Physiology
A Clinical Approach

Physiology
A CLINICAL APPROACH

G. R. Kelman
M.D., Ph.D., M.R.C.P.(Ed.)
Formerly Professor of Human Physiology,
University of Aberdeen

with Chapters 14 and 15 by
T. J. Crow
Ph.D., F.R.C.P.(U.K.), M.R.C.Psych.
Head, Division of Psychiatry,
M.R.C. Clinical Research Centre
Northwick Park Hospital

THIRD EDITION

CHURCHILL LIVINGSTONE
EDINBURGH LONDON MELBOURNE AND NEW YORK 1980

CHURCHILL LIVINGSTONE
Medical Division of Longman Group Limited

Distributed in the United States of America by
Churchill Livingstone Inc., 19 West 44th Street, New
York, N.Y. 10036, and by associated companies,
branches and representatives throughout the world.

First edition 1972
Second edition 1975
Third edition 1980

ISBN 0 443 01820 0

British Library Cataloguing in Publication Data
Kelman, George Richard
    Physiology. - 3rd ed. -
    (Churchill Livingstone medical texts).
    1. Physiology, Pathological
    I. Title
    616.07   RB113   80-41125

Printed in Singapore by Singapore Offset Printing Pte Ltd

Preface to the Third Edition

The need for a new edition of any book means unwelcome work for the author; but, at the same time, is encouraging because it indicates that the previous edition has sold well. And the sale of some thousands of copies of *Physiology: A Clinical Approach* must mean that we are gradually breaking down the undesirable and artificial barrier which still separates physiology and medicine in most medical schools.

Much of the revision work for this new edition has been relatively minor because there have been few if any quantal jumps in our understanding of organ failure during the last five years; but there has been steady progress on several fronts, and I have tried to include most of this new material: for example on hypertension, on the treatment of renal failure, and on our knowledge of haemostatic mechanisms. I have also added a chapter on failure of temperature regulation—fever, hyperthermia and hypothermia—because fever is one of the commonest clinical signs of disease, while hypothermia (which still kills a few healthy individuals each year in the Scottish mountains) is being increasingly recognized as an important cause of morbidity in the elderly.

The conversion to SI units is now almost complete, although I see no reason to change my opinion of the kilo pascal (see Preface to the Second Edition).

I am especially grateful to Dr H. Thurston, Reader in Medicine in the University of Leicester, for his help in revising the chapter on hypertension.

Leicester, 1980   G.R.K.

Preface to the Second Edition

I am naturally pleased that the first edition of this little book has sold well, and that it has become necessary to produce a second edition after a relatively short time. This has permitted me to add new material, including a chapter on defective endocrine function, to clarify and expand various points which were not well expressed in the first edition, and to include certain recent advances, e.g. new knowledge on vitamin D metabolism.

Reviewers have been kind to the first edition; and most people have understood the aim of the book. For the benefit of those who have not let me repeat: the book does not aim to be a comprehensive account either of academic physiology or of clinical medicine—it is obviously far too short for either of these purposes—but it does aim to illuminate the grey area which separates 'preclinical' physiology and 'clinical' subjects, such as medicine and surgery. The physiology section is of necessity somewhat condensed, and will be fully comprehensible only to those who already know some basic physiology; similarly the clinical section will be fully comprehensible only to those who have some acquaintance with clinical medicine and its terminology. Thus, the book is aimed primarily at medical students in the middle years of their course, and at postgraduates working towards the FRCS and MRCP examinations. I hope that it may be of interest also to non-medically qualified 'preclinical' teachers, and to senior science students.

One change in this new edition is the tentative introduction of SI units. The situation as regards these units in medicine at the moment is confused; but I have tried to adopt a common-sense approach, albeit inevitably with the loss of some scientific rigour. The units used here to express routine blood counts are those used by the University of Aberdeen; these are not truly SI units, but have the advantage of keeping the *numbers* the same as those with which we are all familiar, e.g. haemoglobin concentration 15g/dl not 150g/l. I have not adopted the foolishness of using the kilo pascal for blood gas tensions, but have continued to use mmHg—and until blood pressures in the wards are also regularly measured in SI units I shall continue to do so.

In keeping with my original concept of a book which dealt in the main with organ failure, I have limited the endocrine chapter to examples of endocrine hyposecretion, and have not discussed endocrine overactivity at any length.

I am grateful to Mr J. N. Norman, Reader in Surgery, University of Aberdeen for explaining some of the complex electrolyte derangements which accompany chronic pyloric stenosis.

Aberdeen, 1975   G.R.K.

Preface to the First Edition

As physiological and biochemical knowledge advances, the term 'organ failure' is being increasingly heard in hospital wards, both medical and surgical. This concept is a valuable one because the clinical manifestations of impaired function in any given organ tend to be independent of the etiological event which has caused the organ to fail; while treatment must often be directed towards amelioration of the patient's physiological disturbances, rather than towards reversing a well-defined pathological process.

My initial idea for this book was that it would consist of a series of essays describing the physiological basis of the manifestations of various types of organ failure—renal failure, respiratory failure, cardiac failure, peripheral circulatory failure, and so on. I have, however, extended its scope beyond this original idea to include the pathophysiology of certain common signs and symptoms, such as jaundice and oedema, the understanding of which involves a sound knowledge of modern physiology.

My basic viewpoint is that to understand much of modern medicine it is necessary to have a fairly detailed knowledge of physiology, because the present-day tendency is to treat clinical problems from the point of view of disturbed physiology, rather than (as in the past) from the point of view of disturbed anatomy—in terms of 'morbid physiology', rather than of 'morbid anatomy'.

The book is directed primarily at two sets of readers: (a) medical students who are coming towards the end of their physiology course, in which case it aims to show them the relevance of their (perhaps unfortunately named) preclinical studies to their future clinical work, and (b) clinical students, in the hope that it will encourage them to approach clinical problems in a more analytical manner, while at the same time reminding them of certain aspects of their preclinical studies which they may have forgotten. It is hoped also that the book will prove of value to trainee physicians preparing for the MRCP examination.

I am especially grateful to Dr T. J. Crow for writing Chapters 13 and 14. His training in neurophysiology and neuropharmacology, coupled with his clinical expertise, made him a natural choice when I was seeking someone to explain the complex interrelationships between basic neurophysiology and clinical neurology and psychiatry, which form the subject matter of these two chapters.

Aberdeen, 1972   G.R.K.

Contents

Contents

1

Heart failure

The function of the heart is to pump blood round the body, and thus to supply its various tissues with the oxygen and other essential nutrients which they require for their metabolic processes. Heart failure may therefore be said to exist when the output of the heart (the cardiac output, i.e. the amount of blood pumped by the left ventricle each minute) becomes insufficient to supply the body's metabolic requirements.

In order to exclude inadequate tissue perfusion occurring as the result of a reduction of cardiac filling pressure (see Chapter 2), it is customary to exclude from the definition of heart failure a reduction of cardiac output consequent on underfilling of the peripheral circulation. The most convenient definition is therefore probably that of Paul Wood—that heart failure is: 'A state in which the heart fails to maintain an adequate circulation for the needs of the body despite a satisfactory venous filling pressure.'

Heart failure may be acute, as when the functional efficiency of the cardiac pump is suddenly reduced by a myocardial infarction or by a sudden, intolerable load, such as that imposed by a large pulmonary embolus. Or it may be chronic, as when the heart gradually becomes unable to support an increased load which has been present over a considerable period of time. The manifestations of these two conditions differ somewhat: acute heart failure gives rise to the shock syndrome (see next chapter); chronic failure produces the variety of signs and symptoms which are considered later in the present chapter.

In a normal person the output of the heart is able to increase when the tissues' metabolic requirements are increased, as during exercise. When its functional ability is impaired, however, the heart may be able to provide a satisfactory output when the body is at rest, but may be unable to respond adequately when there is a need for increased tissue perfusion. A patient with a mild defect of cardiac function may therefore show the manifestations of failure only during exercise; but, as the condition progresses, symptoms of failure are brought on by progressively less and less exertion, until finally they are present at rest.

1

PHYSIOLOGY

Myocardial contraction

The function of the heart is to convert the chemical potential energy of various complex organic molecules into the mechanical energy possessed by the blood as it flows along the aorta and through the various peripheral tissues. The heart is reasonably omnivorous, and can metabolize a variety of substrates, including fatty acids, glucose, lactate, pyruvate and ketone bodies, roughly in proportion to their relative concentrations in the blood.

As in skeletal muscle, the link between the biochemical breakdown of these complex molecules and the mechanical contraction of the myocardial fibres is provided by the high energy phosphate bonds of adenosine triphosphate (ATP). The energy released by the breakdown of these bonds causes the myocardial contractile proteins (actin and myosin) to undergo a complex physiochemical interaction which results in shortening of the muscle fibres.

The contraction process is initiated by a wave of electrical depolarization of the myocardial membrane. This process commences in the sinoatrial node, and then spreads centrifugally throughout the atria, the atrioventricular node, the bundles of His and the Purkinje* tissue to the right and left ventricles. Calcium ions are involved in coupling membrane depolarization with the actual contraction of the myocardial proteins; but the precise role played by this ion has yet to be defined.

The rhythmic contraction and relaxation of the myocardial muscle, in conjunction with the heart's system of competent oneway valves, causes a unidirectional flow of blood through the heart. The amount of blood which passes through the heart each minute—the cardiac output—depends on both the contractile ability of the myocardium and on the state of the peripheral circulation (see next chapter). The force with which a given region of myocardium contracts depends on its biochemical environment, and on the degree to which it is stretched at the beginning of diastole (Starling's law—see below).

During diastole, blood flows into the relaxed atria and ventricles, gradually distending them to an extent which depends on the pressure in the venous reservoir and on the distensibility of the relaxed myocardium. Atrial contraction at the end of ventricular diastole then forces an additional quantity of blood into the ventricles in preparation for ventricular systole.

(At rest, the main function of the atria is to act as reservoirs which store blood during ventricular systole, ready to pour it into the relaxed

*Correctly spelt Purkyne—Jan Purkyne, Bohemian physiologist 1787-1869.

ventricles when the atrioventricular valves open at the start of ventricular diastole. In exercise, however, atrial contraction probably causes a significant increase of cardiac output, i.e. these appendages then act in a manner rather analogous to a supercharger on an internal combustion engine.)

Ventricular contraction causes the heart to expel blood which has accumulated during diastole into the arterial reservoirs, formed by the pulmonary artery and aorta and their large branches. Ventricular ejection ceases when the pressure in the arterial reservoir exceeds the pressure which can be generated by ventricular contraction.

Starling's law

Cardiac muscle, in common with skeletal muscle, has the property that, the greater its length immediately before the start of contraction, the greater is the force generated when it does contract. This is Starling's law of the heart, which was originally stated in the following terms: 'The law of the heart is thus the same as the law of muscular tissue generally that the energy of contraction, however measured, is a function of the length of the muscle fibre.'

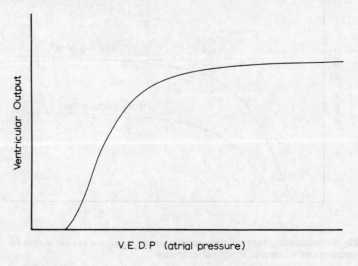

Fig. 1. Relationship between ventricular end-diastolic pressure (V.E.D.P.) and ventricular output.

As a result of this fundamental property of cardiac muscle, the greater the pressure inside the ventricle at the end of diastole (or strictly the greater the pressure differential between the inside of the heart and the surrounding intrathoracic pressure, since it is the pressure differential rather than the absolute intracardiac pressure which distends the heart in diastole), the greater is the amount of blood ejected during its subsequent systole. Thus in the whole heart there is a fairly well-defined functional relationship between ventricular end-diastolic pressure and ventricular output (Fig. 1). And, since ventricular end-diastolic pressure is determined, to a large extent, by the pressure in the appropriate atrium and its associated veins the abscissa in Figure 1 can, with little inaccuracy, be relabelled atrial pressure.

Moreover, also as a result of this law, there is for any given state of cardiac functional efficiency a well-defined experimental relationship between *right* atrial pressure (r.a.p., which is measured clinically as central venous pressure-q.v.) and the output of the *left* ventricle (cardiac output), as shown in Figure 2. (The reason for this perhaps unexpected finding is that an increase of r.a.p. increases the output of the right ventricle, thus increasing the amount of blood in the pulmonary circulation, and therefore the filling pressure of the left ventricle, and so by Starling's law causing an increase in left ventricu-

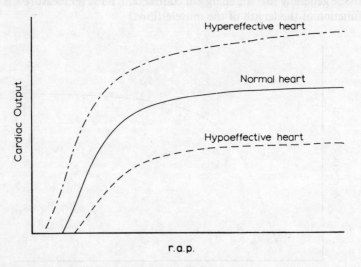

Fig. 2. Relationship between right atrial pressure (r.a.p.) and cardiac output for several states of cardiac functional efficiency.

lar output.) Cardiac output increases with increasing values of r.a.p. until, at high atrial pressures, it tends to become constant.

It is perhaps worth noting that Starling's original curves tended to show a decrease of cardiac output at very high cardiac filling pressures. More recent work, however, has suggested that this fall of output was an artefact due to non-specific deterioration of the isolated heart-lung preparation which he used. It may also be however that high distending pressures stretch the valve rings of the atrioventricular valves, thus causing their functional incompetence and a consequent decline of cardiac output (see p. 7).

The solid curve in Figure 2 refers to a heart in which myocardial contractility and valvular competence are normal, and in which there is consequently a normal relationship between r.a.p. and cardiac output. Under these circumstances the normal cardiac output of about 5 1/min occurs at a transmural right atrial pressure of a few cmH_2O. (In man the normal central venous pressure lies in the range 6 to 12 cmH_2O.)

Myocardial contractility, i.e. the ability of the cardiac muscle to contract and generate a mechanical force, varies in response to different physiological stimuli, and in pathological states. An alteration in this parameter results in a change of cardiac efficiency, and therefore in the position of the curve relating cardiac output and r.a.p. Cardiac functional efficiency may also be altered by disease processes which impair the functional competence of the cardiac valves.

The upper curve in Figure 2 represents a hypereffective heart, in which myocardial contractility is increased, as might occur, for example, under the influence of sympathetic stimulation or increased adrenal catecholamine secretion. Such a heart can provide an above-normal cardiac output at a given r.a.p. or, what amounts to the same thing, can achieve a normal cardiac output at a subnormal filling pressure.

The lower curve in Figure 2 represents a hypoeffective heart, such as might occur as a result of myocardial hypoxia or ischaemia, or damage to a cardiac valve. In this case a normal cardiac output can be achieved only at a filling pressure which is above normal. Blood is therefore dammed back in the venous circulation, and it is this increase of pressure behind the failing heart which is responsible for many of the clinical manifestations of heart failure, e.g. pulmonary oedema when the functional defect affects predominantly the left side of the heart, and systemic oedema with distended neck veins and an enlarged, tender liver when cardiac function is impaired as a whole.

PATHOPHYSIOLOGY

Acute heart failure

A sudden reduction of cardiac efficiency, as by a myocardial infarction or pulmonary embolus, causes the heart to become a less satisfactory pump than previously. The cardiac function curve therefore becomes depressed, and the output which can be achieved at a given r.a.p. is reduced, while maintenance of a normal output requires a greater than normal cardiac filling pressure.

The net result is a reduction of cardiac output and a rise of r.a.p.; but this situation is modified by the body's compensatory mechanisms in the following way. For reasons considered in the section on shock (q.v.) an acute reduction of cardiac output acts via the carotid and aortic baroreceptors to cause increased efferent sympathetic activity to the heart and other regions of the cardiovascular system. Increased cardiac sympathetic drive increases myocardial contractility and therefore the efficiency of the cardiac pump, so moving the cardiac function curve upwards and to the left towards its normal position. At the same time constriction of the veins tends to raise the cardiac filling pressure and, in conjunction with improved myocardial contractility, restores cardiac output towards normal.

The typical response of the body to an acute reduction of cardiac efficiency is thus a reduction of cardiac output (but not to the extent which would occur in the absence of compensatory mechanisms), accompanied by an increase of r.a.p. due partly to depression of cardiac function and partly to the venoconstriction which accompanies an increase of sympathetic activity.

At the same time, increased sympathetic activity causes constriction of the peripheral resistance vessels (see section on hypertension) in various tissues, and redirects blood from less vital organs, such as the kidney, gut and skin, towards more immediately essential organs, such as the heart and brain (see section on shock).

Of course, certain disease processes tend to affect predominantly the function of one or other side of the heart, rather than to cause a generalized decrease of cardiac functional efficiency as discussed above. When the defect is confined mainly to the left side of the heart, as it often is in the case of a myocardial infarction, the increase of cardiac filling pressure occurs predominantly in the left atrium. (In patients with an intact pericardium, however, an increase of left atrial pressure, due, for example, to left ventricular dysfunction, is usually accompanied by increased strain on the *right* ventricle, and therefore by an increase of r.a.p. This may not be the case in patients in whom the pericardium is congenitally absent, or in whom it has been removed at operation. In such circumstances r.a.p. may be a poor guide to the pressures in the pulmonary circulation.)

Chronic heart failure

In chronic heart failure the functional efficiency of the cardiac pump is reduced, therefore (for reasons considered above) the patient has a reduced cardiac output and an increased r.a.p. In addition, the body responds to the altered haemodynamic state by retention of water and electrolytes (chiefly sodium), causing marked expansion of the extra-cellular fluid volume (see section on oedema). By increasing cardiac filling pressure, this fluid retention probably helps to maintain an adequate cardiac output; but ultimately it may become excessive, with the result that symptoms due to fluid retention become as troublesome to the patient as those due directly to his reduced cardiac output.

Also, if the increase of venous pressure is too great, diastolic distension of the right ventricle may become so marked that incompetence of the tricuspid valve develops, causing a further decrease of cardiac functional efficiency.

In acute heart failure the cause of the reduced cardiac efficiency is usually obvious enough; but in chronic failure the etiology of the condition is sometimes obscure. In chronic myocardial ischaemia due to coronary artery disease, defective cardiac function is clearly the result of myocardial hypoxia, and indeed, under these circumstances, the myocardial muscle may be partially replaced by non-contractile fibrous tissue; but in other conditions, such as chronic valvular disease, the cause of the defective cardiac function is often less clear.

When a chronically increased load is imposed on the heart—as by arterial hypertension, a valvular defect, or by a reduction of the oxygen carrying capacity of the blood (see section on anaemia)—the heart is initially able to increase its pumping efficiency by myocardial hyper-trophy. As a result, the body is able to compensate initially for the increased load; sooner or later, however, and for reasons which are rather unclear, the heart becomes unable to maintain a cardiac output sufficient for the needs of the body. Chronic heart failure has then developed.

The fundamental defect in chronic cardiac failure seems to be an abnormality of the actual myocardial contractile proteins, actin and myosin. Energy liberation and energy storage appear to be normal. The precise physicochemical nature of the defect of contraction is, however, unknown, although it is said that the contractility of actomy-osin bands taken from patients dying of congestive cardiac failure is impaired, and may be partially restored by the addition of digoxin. Also, there is some evidence that calcium transfer through the myocardial membrane may be reduced, suggesting that the failing heart has a defect of excitation-contraction coupling.

Haemodynamics in chronic failure
The resting cardiac output of patients with moderate or severe chronic heart failure is reduced below the normal value of 5 1/min, sometimes markedly so. As a result, certain tissues, such as the kidneys, the gut,

and the limbs are starved of blood, and many of the symptoms of chronic heart failure, such as fluid retention, anorexia, nausea and vomiting, and fatigue are due to impaired perfusion of peripheral tissues. The arterioles and other resistance vessels in such underperfused tissues are constricted, therefore the resistance to blood flow around the body (total peripheral resistance) is increased, and the reduced cardiac output is accompanied by an almost normal arterial blood pressure. (Mean arterial blood pressure is, to a first approximation, equal to the product of cardiac output and total peripheral resistance—see section on hypertension.)

In patients with relatively mild failure, cardiac output may be normal at rest, but fails to increase adequately in response to the increased metabolic requirements of exercise. In severe failure, cardiac output may be markedly reduced at rest, and increases little, or not at all, during exercise. This disparity between cardiac output and the body's metabolic requirements is reflected in the oxygen content of the mixed-venous blood. In chronic failure the oxygen saturation of the blood returning to the right side of the heart is lower than normal; and this fact, in conjunction with the reduced cardiac output, results in a marked reduction (up to 50 per cent) in the amount of oxygen returning each minute to the heart, and therefore in the oxygen reserve available to the body. (It should be noted, however, that the correlation between the severity of a patient's failure, as assessed in this way, and the severity of his symptoms is poor, a situation reminiscent of that found in chronic anaemia.)

High output heart failure
In certain conditions the body's metabolic requirements are such that cardiac output must be considerably increased if tissue metabolism is to proceed normally. This is the case, for example, in thyrotoxicosis, and when the peripheral haemoglobin concentration is reduced by anaemia (q.v.). Both these conditions impose a chronically increased load on the heart, and may ultimately result in cardiac failure. When this happens, cardiac output is reduced, and although it may still be above normal, symptoms of failure become evident. This is the condition of high output cardiac failure, in which the output of the heart, although above normal, is reduced below the level appropriate to the body's increased metabolic needs.

Fluid retention
One of the most noticeable features of chronic heart failure is a marked increase of extracellular fluid volume. This expansion is due partly to an increased red cell mass (presumably secondary to chronic hypoxia

of the bone marrow), but still more to sodium and water retention occurring as a result of impaired renal function (see section on sodium balance).

Although patients with chronic heart failure usually have decreased renal blood flow and glomerular filtration rates, their primary renal defect appears to be excessive tubular reabsorption of sodium and water, rather than decreased filtration of these substances by the glomerular capillaries. This increased sodium reabsorption is probably the result of increased aldosterone activity with enhanced sodium/potassium exchange across the walls of the distal convoluted tubules (see chapter on renal failure). The reason for such excessive aldosterone secretion is uncertain; it is probably due, in part, to overactivity of the renin-angiotensin system (see section on hypertension) in response to a chronic reduction of renal blood flow.

CLINICAL MANIFESTATIONS OF HEART FAILURE

The clinical manifestations of acute heart failure are considered in the next chapter.

In the past it was customary to divide the clinical manifestations of chronic heart failure into signs and symptoms which were thought to be due to 'forward failure', i.e. to the fact that cardiac output is below normal, and into signs and symptoms due to 'backward failure', i.e. manifestations which are the result of increased venous pressure behind the failing heart. It is now apparent, however, that much of the venous congestion and peripheral oedema of chronic heart failure arises not so much from the increased venous pressure *per se*, as from the water and electrolyte retention which accompanies a chronic reduction of cardiac efficiency. Thus, although the division into forward failure and backward failure may at times be convenient, it tends to impair understanding of the pathogenesis of the manifestations of cardiac failure and is therefore probably best avoided.

It is also convenient to divide the clinical manifestations of heart failure into those which are due predominantly to left-sided failure, and those which are due mainly to right-sided failure. It must be remembered, however, that both sides of the heart are often simultaneously affected by disease, and both sides may fail together—the condition of congestive cardiac failure. Further, left-sided failure causes a marked rise of pressure in the pulmonary circulation, thus imposing a considerable strain on the right side of the heart, ultimately causing it to fail. The commonest cause of right-sided heart failure is pre-existing left-sided failure.

Patients with both types of heart failure show signs of inadequate peripheral perfusion with cyanosis of the extremities, ready fatigability and lack of energy. They may complain also of abdominal symptoms, such as anorexia, nausea and vomiting, which are due to inadequate gastrointestinal blood flow. Such symptoms may be confused with the effects of digitalis over-dosage.

Left-sided failure

Failure predominantly of the left side of the heart occurs in patients with systemic hypertension (q.v.), aortic valvular disease and coronary atheroma. The essential symptom of left-sides heart failure is dyspnoea—excessive shortness of breath—on exercise, or even at rest. This symptom arises as a result of pulmonary congestion, which causes a reduction of pulmonary compliance, and therefore increases the muscular effort required to move air in and out of the lungs (see section on respiratory failure). Increased pulmonary venous pressure may also cause a troublesome cough, sometimes with haemoptysis due to rupture of congested pulmonary capillaries.

At first the dyspnoea of cardiac failure occurs only during exercise; as the condition progresses, however, the symptom is provoked by less and less exertion, until finally it is present at rest. Many patients exhibit orthopnoea, that is they become dyspnoeic only on lying down. This symptom appears to be due partly to the fact that the recumbent position impedes diaphragmatic movement, and partly to the fact that, in this position, blood is transferred from the normally dependent parts of the body to the pulmonary circulation, where it enhances the already-present congestion. In addition, patients may experience nocturnal paroxysms of dyspnoea, in which they are awakened from sleep by intense shortness of breath, which is relieved by getting up and assuming the upright position. Such patients may also wheeze— the condition of cardiac asthma.

The pressure in the pulmonary circulation is normally only about one-fifth as great as that in the systemic circulation. The tendency for fluid to leave the pulmonary capillaries is correspondingly reduced; and the lungs are readily kept 'dry' by the oncotic pressure of the plasma proteins (about 25 mmHg—see section on oedema). When the hydrostatic pressure in the pulmonary capillaries is raised, however, fluid is forced out of the capillaries into the pulmonary alveoli, where it impedes the uptake of oxygen, and, to a lesser extent, the elimination of carbon dioxide. This is the condition of pulmonary oedema, a serious complication of left-sided failure, which, if not energetically treated, may be rapidly fatal.

Examination of the lungs of a patient with left-sided failure reveals the presence of moist, adventitious sounds in the form of basal crepitations of all grades of severity. The heart is enlarged, and in addition to possible murmurs from causative valvular lesions, auscultation may reveal an abnormal third heart sound, which probably arises from rapid ventricular filling as a result of the high cardiac filling pressure. When, as is usually the case, the heart beat is rapid, the three heart sounds take on a characteristic cadence known as gallop rhythm, a sign of considerable diagnostic importance.

Right heart failure

The commonest causes of right heart failure are preceding left-sided failure and chronic lung disease with pulmonary hypertension (q.v.). Dyspnoea is not a prominent feature of right-sided failure unless it is associated with chronic lung disease. In fact, the paroxysmal nocturnal dyspnoea of left-sided failure may be considerably improved when right-sided failure supervenes; pulmonary congestion is thereby relieved, giving the patient a false impression that he is getting better.

In right-sided failure there is considerable engorgement of the systemic circulation, with distended neck veins and an enlarged, tender liver. Such distension is best seen in the internal jugular vein, because the external jugular is commonly kinked by the cervical fascia. The height of the pressure in the right atrium may be estimated clinically by measuring the height to which the jugular venous column of blood rises above the sternal angle with the patient partially sitting up.

Patients with right-sided failure usually have oedema of the peripheral, dependent parts of the body. This is due partly to the raised venous pressure, but probably more to the marked retention of water and electrolytes which accompanies this condition (see earlier). There may also be frank accumulations of fluid in the body's serous cavities, with hydrothorax, pericardial effusion and ascites. A small proportion of patients develop cirrhosis of the liver (q.v.) from chronic hepatic congestion.

PHYSIOLOGICAL PRINCIPLES OF TREATMENT

The treatment of heart failure rests firmly on three foundations: appropriate limitation of physical exertion, administration of digitalis glycosides and of diuretics to promote sodium and water excretion by the kidneys—to rid the body of excess extracellular fluid (see earlier). In a few cases, of course, it is possible to treat the primary cause of the failure: anaemia, some forms of congenital heart disease and thyrotoxicosis are obvious examples. But in most cases treatment must be symptomatic only.

Digitalis increases the force of contraction of the failing myocardium. Its precise mode of action is unknown, but is thought to be related to its effects on intracellular calcium. Digitalis increases the intracellular calcium ion concentration, perhaps by inhibiting the myocardial sodium pump; it also prevents calcium uptake by the cytoplasmic reticulum. The resulting increase of intracellular calcium availability increases the force of myocardial contraction, without, it is said, increasing its oxygen consumption (cf. the action of the sympathomimetic amines which increase myocardial contractility but only at the expense of increased oxygen consumption).

In addition, digitalis slows the heart rate both by a direct action on the conducting tissues, and indirectly via the vagus. It also increases myocardial excitability—a side effect which may lead to troublesome, or even fatal, arrhythmias: ventricular extrasystoles, coupled beats (pulsus bigeminus) and ventricular tachycardia or even fibrillation. These toxic effects may be enhanced by hypokalaemia as a result of diuretic therapy (see below).

The administration of diuretics increases the renal excretion of sodium and water, and thus removes the excessive accumulations of extracellular fluid which are responsible for many of the clinical manifestations of cardiac failure, e.g. systemic and pulmonary oedema. Many diuretics, particularly the thiazides and frusemide, tend to cause potassium depletion, which must be prevented by the administration of dietary potassium supplements. This increased potassium loss appears to arise mainly as a result of the action of these diuretics on the proximal renal tubules where they reduce sodium reabsorption (see Chapter 7); the resulting increased sodium load reaching the distal tubules causes excessive sodium/potassium exchange (under the influence of aldosterone) with a resulting increase in urinary potassium excretion. This is particularly the case when there is increased aldosterone activity, as there may be if the diuresis is sufficient to cause extracellular fluid depletion.

Digitalis itself causes a diuresis. This is mainly the result of its action in improving the peripheral circulation and so increasing renal blood flow; but is also by a direct effect on the renal tubules.

FURTHER READING

Anon 1978 Vasodilators in heart failure. Lancet i: 972
Anon 1978 Imbalanced ventricles and cardiac failure. British Medical Journal i: 324
Anon 1979 Treatments for heart-failure: stimulation of unloading. Lancet ii: 777
Arnott W M 1966 Heart failure. British Medical Journal ii: 1585

Braunwald E 1979 Heart failure. In: Harper R S, Muir J P (eds) Advanced medicine 15. Pitman Medical, Tunbridge Wells

Campbell E J M, Dickinson C J, Slater J D H 1974 Clinical physiology, 4th edn. Blackwell, Oxford, ch 2

Guyton A C 1963 Cardiac output and its regulation, 2nd edn. Saunders, Philadelphia

Henderson A H 1975 Contractile basis of heart failure. In: Oliver M F Modern trends in cardiology, 3rd edn. Butterworths, London, ch 7

Kelman G R 1977 Applied cardiovascular physiology, 2nd edn. Butterworths, London, ch 2

McKendrick C S 1967 Recognition of heart failure. British Medical Journal ii: 219

Myerson R M, Pastor B H 1967 Congestive heart failure. C V Mosby, St Louis

Rushmer R F 1970 Cardiovascular dynamics, 3rd edn. Saunders, Philadelphia

Towers M K 1966 Chronic cor pulmonale. Post-Graduate Medical Journal 42: 506

Wood P 1968 Diseases of the heart and circulation, 3rd edn. Eyre & Spottiswoode, London, ch 7

Zelis R, Longhurst J 1975 The circulation in congestive heart failure. In: Zelis R (ed) The peripheral circulations. Grune and Stratton, New York, ch 13

2

Shock and peripheral circulatory failure

The clinical syndrome known as shock * is more easily recognized than described. A patient suffering from this condition presents a characteristic appearance: he has a pale, anxious, sweating and often slightly cyanosed countenance, coupled with a greater or lesser degree of prostration, and often with some clouding of consciousness. Although one of the commonest causes of shock is hypovolaemia, the shock syndrome is not confined to surgical wards and operating theatres; it occurs also in medical wards in such conditions as myocardial infarction and acute adrenal insufficiency (q.v.).

Although one of the important signs of shock is a reduction of arterial blood pressure, there is much to be said for considering the primary physiological defect in this condition to be a reduction of cardiac output and therefore of total body perfusion, rather than a reduction of arterial pressure *per se*. Indeed, a previously hypertensive patient may show the manifestations of shock in the presence of an arterial blood pressure which is not outside the normal range. Further, injudicious attempts to raise the blood pressure of shocked patients by giving alpha-stimulating sympathomimetic amines may increase the strain on a heart which has been damaged by hypoxia, ischaemia, etc., and may therefore result in a paradoxical worsening of the patient's clinical condition. The most convenient definition is thus that of Guyton who defines shock as 'a state of the circulation in which tissues in widespread areas of the body are being damaged by nutritive insufficiency resulting from inadequate cardiac output'.

Despite this definition, it is now being increasingly recognized that some patients who clinically appear shocked, have cardiac outputs which are within the normal range. These patients often have severe bacterial infections, particularly in association with hepatic cirrhosis; and it appears that, in many cases, they have abnormal vascular channels through which blood can pass from the arterial to the venous

*Not to be confused with psychological or emotional shock which may induce a vasovagal (fainting) attack and a short-lived hypotensive episode which, however, recovers rapidly and spontaneously.

14

sides of the circulation without passing through the tissue capillaries. Under these circumstances tissue perfusion may be inadequate for the needs of the body even though the cardiac output is normal, or even above normal.

Clinical experience shows that the shock syndrome may occur in two main groups of patients. On the one hand, there are those in whom the syndrome is due to a defect of cardiac function—cardiogenic shock; on the other hand, there are the patients in whom the peripheral circulation is underfilled with blood so that their cardiac filling pressure is inadequate to maintain a satisfactory cardiac output—peripheral circulatory failure. The commonest cause of the former condition is myocardial infarction; the commonest (and most easily treated) cause of the latter is acute hypovolaemia due to trauma.

PHYSIOLOGY

Regulation of cardiac output

In order to understand the pathogenesis of the shock syndrome it is essential to have a clear understanding of the way in which the body regulates its cardiac output. Confusion is caused by failure to realize that cardiac output depends on the interplay of two factors: the pumping ability of the heart and the state of the peripheral circulation. Such confusion is not helped by statements of the kind: 'In haemorrhage, cardiac output is low because venous return is reduced.' Since the heart and peripheral circulation are connected in series, the venous return (the amount of blood flowing back to the right side of the heart each minute) must, over any appreciable period of time, equal the cardiac output (the amount of blood leaving the left ventricle each minute). What the statement really means of course is that the state of the peripheral circulation is such that the pressure available to cause blood to flow back to the heart is reduced, and, as a result, cardiac output is reduced.

Right atrial pressure

Central to any account of the regulation of cardiac output is an apreciation of the role played by the right atrial pressure (r.a.p.). As discussed in Chapter 1, an increase of r.a.p. causes, by the Starling mechanism, an increase of cardiac output. But, at the same time, an increase of r.a.p. tends to dam blood back in the peripheral circulation, and thus to reduce the rate at which it can flow back into the heart— the venous return. But venous return equals cardiac output, therefore there is the paradoxical situation that an increase of r.a.p. is accompanied simultaneously by an *increase* of cardiac output and by a *decrease* of venous return which is equal to cardiac output.

The solution to this paradox lies in the fact that the body adjusts its r.a.p. at such a level that the rate of blood flow onwards through the heart is just equal to the rate of blood flow back into the heart from the great veins. If the venous return momentarily exceeds the cardiac output, r.a.p. rises until cardiac *input* (venous return) and cardiac output are once again in balance.

A decrease in the pumping efficiency of the heart means that this organ can expel a given cardiac output only at a higher than normal r.a.p. (see previous chapter). Blood is therefore dammed back in the large veins, and in consequence right atrial pressure rises until it is again at such a level that the (reduced) venous return is just equal to the (reduced) cardiac output. The body comes to a new equilibrium with a higher than normal r.a.p. and a lower than normal cardiac output.

A reduction in the amount of blood in the peripheral circulation causes a decrease in the pressures which are available there to force blood back to the heart. (Guyton calls the resultant of these peripheral pressures the 'mean systemic pressure': a valuable, but somewhat complicated concept—see recommended further reading). Venous return can then be maintained only if r.a.p. falls until the body is once again in equilibrium, with venous return equal to cardiac output, but with a low r.a.p. and a lower than normal cardiac output.

Physiological response to a reduction of cardiac output

The mean blood pressure in the aorta and its large branches is, to a first approximation, proportional to the product of cardiac output and the total resistance to blood flow presented by all the body's peripheral tissues connected in parallel between the aorta and the venae cavae. This total resistance is called the 'total peripheral resistance'—see next chapter. A reduction of cardiac output thus tends to cause a reduction of mean arterial pressure, and this fall of pressure is detected by the aortic and carotid baroreceptors, so inducing a variety of compensatory mechanisms which tend to restore cardiac output and arterial pressure towards normal (see below).

The decreased afferent activity which passes to the medullary cardiovascular 'centres'* as a result of a decrease of arterial pressure causes an increase of efferent sympathetic activity to the whole

---

*It is now believed that the medullary centres are not anatomically discrete collections of neurones, and that the cardiovascular reflex pathways pass not only through the medulla but also through higher centres.

cardiovascular system and to the adrenal medullae. The adrenal hormones, adrenaline and noradrenaline, liberated in response to such stimulation reinforce the effects of the generalized increase of sympathetic activity.

(A similar response may occur even when the mean arterial pressure is not greatly reduced. Cardiovascular stress is usually accompanied by a reduction of cardiac stroke volume, and this in turn moves the systolic and diastolic arterial pressures closer together, and therefore reduces the arterial pulse pressure. It is known that the baroreceptors are sensitive not only to mean pressure, but also to rate of change of pressure; they therefore respond not only to a reduction of mean arterial pressure, but also to a reduction of pulse pressure.)

Increased efferent sympathetic activity to the heart causes an increase of myocardial contractility (see previous chapter), thus increasing the cardiac output which can be produced at a given r.a.p. The extent to which increased sympathetic drive can increase the functional efficiency of the cardiac pump clearly depends on the pre-existing state of the myocardium—the response of a heart severely damaged by myocardial infarction is likely to be less satisfactory than that of a heart in which the myocardium is normal. Increased efferent sympathetic activity also causes constriction of the peripheral veins, thus tending to increase the pressure available to drive blood back to the heart (Guyton's mean systemic pressure). As a result, there is a further increase of r.a.p. and cardiac output.

At the same time there is constriction of the peripheral resistance vessels—the arterioles, metarterioles, and precapillary sphincters—in a variety of tissues, thus increasing the total peripheral resistance, and restoring the arterial blood pressure towards normal.

Redistribution of cardiac output

Such sympathetically-induced vasoconstriction does not affect all tissues uniformly; a generalized increase of efferent sympathetic activity constricts the vessels in some tissues more than in others. For example, although the blood vessels of the cerebral circulation are anatomically well supplied with sympathetic neurones, this innervation apears to be of little functional significance; a generalized increase of sympathetic activity therefore has little effect on the cerebral vasculature. On the other hand, the blood vessels in other tissues, such as the skin, kidney and gut, are very sensitive to sympathetic stimulation and to circulating catecholamines; they therefore respond to increased sympathetic activity with marked vasoconstriction. As a result, a generalized increase of sympathetic activity diverts blood flow away from tissues, such as the gut and kidney, which (in the short term) are relatively unimportant to the economy of the body, to more immediately essential organs, such as the brain and heart.

As will be seen later, the intense vasoconstriction which occurs in certain tissues may cause complications. Although initially it tends to maintain the arterial blood pressure and the perfusion of vital organs, it deprives other tissues of the blood which they need to maintain their metabolic activity. Ultimately it may damage the ischaemic, hypoxic tissues with potentially lethal consequences to the body as a whole.

PATHOPHYSIOLOGY

It is convenient to categorize cases of shock according to the condition's pathogenesis. It must be remembered however that the various categories are not as mutually exclusive as is sometimes taught; there may, for example, be an element of defective cardiac function (due to ischaemia and metabolic acidosis) in shock primarily due to haemorrhage.

Hypovolaemic shock (peripheral circulatory failure)

A reduction in the amount of blood contained in the peripheral circulation reduces the pressure available there to return blood to the heart, and causes a reduction of both r.a.p. and cardiac output (see earlier). This is an example of hypovolaemic shock; a condition which may occur also when there is severe loss of extracellular fluid from some other cause (see section on sodium depletion). The same situation may occur even when the blood volume is normal if the capacity of the peripheral circulation is increased, as by the action of alpha-blocking sympatholytic drugs, or by the action of circulating bacterial toxins.

Cardiogenic shock

As discussed in a previous section, a generalized reduction in the efficiency of the cardiac pump causes a reduction of cardiac output and a rise of cardiac filling pressure (r.a.p.). This is the condition of cardiogenic shock, as may occur after a severe myocardial infarction.

Also it is thought that many patients, who initially have peripheral circulatory failure, ultimately develop an element of cardiogenic shock, leading to worsening of their clinical condition, and often to death. The cause of this deterioration of cardiac function is uncertain: the heart may be damaged by bacterial toxins, liberated from ischaemic gut or elsewhere; it may be damaged by lactic acid formed by anaerobic metabolism in ischaemic tissues; or the myocardium itself may be rendered ischaemic as a result of arterial hypotension.

Several of these factors may act in concord. Uncorrected metabolic acidosis (q.v.) can cause a severe impairment of cardiac function, and may initiate the vicious circle in which a reduction of cardiac output causes poor perfusion of peripheral tissues, and therefore more acidosis and a further deterioration of cardiac function, ultimately with fatal results.

Septic shock

In addition to the two main types of shock considered above the condition of septic shock is being increasingly recognized. The precise nature of this condition is, however, uncertain, and probably differs from patient to patient. The possibility that patients with septic shock, particularly those in whom this accompanies hepatic cirrhosis, may have abnormal arterio-venous communications has already been mentioned. In addition, bacterial toxins may impair myocardial function, and, by causing venous dilatation, may cause pooling of blood in the peripheral circulation and a reduction of cardiac filling pressure (see earlier). Bacterial toxins may also damage tissue capillaries, allowing plasma to leave the circulation, so causing a reduction of blood volume with an increase of blood viscosity, and peripheral circulatory stagnation. Some patients with this condition appear to have a cardiac output which is above the normal range, but the increased blood flow is diverted away from the body's essential tissues.

Reversible versus irreversible shock

It is customary to classify shock into two categories: reversible and irreversible. Irreversible in this context does not mean untreatable, but merely refers to the fact that restoration of the patient's blood volume to normal does not result in his rapid restoration to health, as it does in a patient with reversible shock. A fit young adult suffering from shock as a result of acute blood loss can be restored to physiological normality simply by restoration of his blood volume. Traumatic shock in an older patient, however, or in a younger patient who has remained in the shocked state for several hours is considerably more resistant to treatment; and the restoration to health of a patient with such 'irreversible shock' presents the physician and clinical physiologist with a complex therapeutic problem which present knowledge is often insufficient to answer—the shock often turns out to be truly irreversible.

Causes of irreversibility

There is evidence that an important factor in determining the irreversibility or otherwise of the shocked state is the condition of the patient's microcirculation—vessels such as the arterioles, metarterioles, capillaries and venules of less than 100 μm in diameter. In severe shock, tissue hypoxia induces paralysis of the vascular smooth muscle surrounding these vessels; but the arterioles and metarterioles appear to become paralysed before the venules, thus causing the capillaries to become overfilled with blood, and allowing plasma to leak out into the interstitial spaces. Blood thus becomes sequestered in the capillaries, and fluid is lost in the interstitial spaces between the tissue cells, causing a marked reduction of functional blood volume. This blood which is trapped in the overfilled capillaries was referred to by Cannon as 'the blood which is out of currency', meaning that, although it had not been lost by external haemorrhage, and was therefore still within the body, it was not available for the carriage of oxygen and other nutrients to the tissues.

Hardaway has suggested that, if the process described in the previous paragraph is not reversed by appropriate treatment, it may result in the capillaries becoming filled with a 'sludge' of erythrocytes, so that such tissue blood flow as persists is forced to bypass the capillaries through arterio-venous communications. If such intravascular sludging is allowed to persist, there may be actual intravascular thrombosis in the vessels of the microcirculation. And it is to ameliorate such intravascular stasis that some workers recommend the administration of low molecular-weight dextran to severely shocked patients; they do so in the hope that, by reducing blood viscosity and the tendency for red cell aggregation, they may be able to improve microcirculatory perfusion.

Central venous pressure (c.v.p.)

It is common clinical practice to estimate the pressure in the right atrium by means of a saline manometer, coupled to a thin, percutaneously-introduced 'central venous catheter', lying with its tip in one of the large intrathoracic veins or in the right atrium itself. The normal range of this 'central venous pressure' (c.v.p.) is somewhat wide, but is usually accepted to lie between 6 and 12 cmH$_2$O, relative to the midaxillary line with the patient in the horizontal position, or to a line directed horizontally backwards from the sternal angle if the patient is not horizontal.

The height of the c.v.p. is of considerable diagnostic importance in establishing the cause of an individual patient's shocked state. For reasons considered earlier, c.v.p. is low when the cardiac output is inadequate as a result of underfilling of the peripheral circulation, and tends to be high when the patient's condition is due primarily to defective cardiac function. (When the abnormality of cardiac function affects predominantly the left ventricle the increase of cardiac filling pressure is mainly on the left side also. It appears, however, that in a patient with an intact pericardium an increase of left artial pressure is accompanied also by an increase of right atrial pressure).

Central venous pressure measurements are particularly valuable as a guide to the adequacy or otherwise of fluid replacement. It is difficult to measure a patient's blood volume accurately, and, even if it were possible to do so, it would be even more difficult to decide if this blood volume was appropriate to the state of his peripheral circulation. If the capacity of a patient's venous reservoir is increased, as by sympatholytic drugs given in the management of irreversible shock (see later), his blood volume may be within the normal range at a time when his c.v.p., and therefore his cardiac output, is severely reduced. Although the blood volume of such a patient is normal, it is not appropriate to the increased capacity of his peripheral circulation; and under these circumstances cardiac output can be restored only by expansion of the blood volume until the cardiac filling pressure is satisfactory, even though this means expanding the blood vol. outside the normal range.

CLINICAL MANIFESTATIONS IN SHOCK

Reduction of blood flow

In the face of an acute reduction of tissue perfusion, the body attempts to redirect the reduced cardiac output towards those tissues which are most essential for its immediate survival. As a result other tissues, such as the skin, kidneys and gut, are rendered ischaemic to a greater or lesser degree; and this ischaemia may ultimately have serious consequences on the affected organs (see section on irreversible shock).

In addition to causing marked pallor, the increased efferent sympathetic activity to the skin causes increased (and inappropriate) sweating, so that the patient feels cold and clammy. And the reduction of renal blood flow leads to marked oliguria, which, if not rapidly reversed by appropriate treatment, may progress to acute tubular necrosis and renal failure (q.v.). Measurement of urine flow rate is a valuable, and somewhat neglected investigation, which may be of considerable help in the management of a shocked patient. Inadequate urine flow in the early stages of shock suggests that, whatever the patient's general appearance, his renal blood flow is considerably below normal, presumably because his cardiac output is reduced. It is thus an indication that further treatment is required.

Reduction of blood pressure

Although, for reasons considered in a later section, decreased arterial blood pressure is of secondary importance in the pathogenesis of the shocked state, it is responsible for many of its clinical manifestations.

The patient's prostration arises from the fact that, except when he is in the horizontal position, his blood pressure is insufficient to pump blood up to his brain against the effects of gravity. Also, a certain intravascular pressure is necessary in the kidney to cause glomerular filtration against the osmotic pressure of the plasma proteins. And in the brain there is a limit to the extent to which autoregulation (see next chapter) can maintain cerebral perfusion in the face of a reduced arterial pressure. (Cerebral autoregulation is probably impaired in patients who have become accustomed to a chronically raised arterial pressure, or whose cerebral vasculature is affected by atheroma. Such patients withstand arterial hypotension badly.)

In the lungs the consequences of the reduction of (pulmonary) arterial pressure are still more important. Even in the normal state, the pulmonary arterial pressure is only about one-fifth that in the systemic circulation. As a result, the upper regions of the lung receive very little blood flow; and, when the pulmonary arterial pressure is reduced by an acute reduction of cardiac output, large regions of lung become almost completely unperfused. The alveoli in these regions do not take part in gas exchange; and they therefore become part of the patient's physiological dead space.

As a result of this increase in physiological dead space, the total pulmonary ventilation (minute volume) required to achieve a given alveolar ventilation is increased (see section on respiratory failure). Shocked patients may therefore show the phenomenon of 'air hunger'—a deep, sighing type of respiration, similar to that seen in metabolic acidosis which may be present as well.

Despite the relative inefficiency of their pulmonary ventilation, however, shocked patients are normally well able to eliminate their metabolically-produced carbon dioxide. The arterial CO_2 tension in shock is, in fact, usually somewhat below normal, although the injudicious administration of narcotic analgesics such as morphine may depress the patient's respiratory centre(s) so that he is no longer able to maintain a sufficient minute volume to overcome his increased physiological dead space. Respiratory failure (q.v.) then develops.

PHYSIOLOGICAL PRINCIPLES OF TREATMENT

Although one of the important signs of shock is a marked reduction of arterial blood pressure, most evidence suggests that it is not the reduction of arterial pressure *per se* which is of central importance in the pathogenesis of the shocked state, but the accompanying reduction of cardiac output. Cannon wrote in 1923: 'Merely a higher arterial pressure is not the desideratum in the treatment of shock, but a higher pressure which provides an increased nutritive flow through the capillaries all over the body'. Treatment must therefore be directed towards increasing the reduced cardiac output, rather than towards restoring the arterial pressure. (Increase of the patient's cardiac output will, however, usually result in a secondary improvement of arterial pressure.)

Treatment of haemorrhagic shock is straightforward unless it has persisted for some hours, thus allowing the condition to become 'irreversible' (see p. 19). Restoration of blood volume in such patients should preferably be guided by measurement of c.v.p., because it is necessary to guide the patient between the Scylla of overtransfusion and the Charybdis of hypovolaemia. Overtransfusion exposes the patient to the risk of pulmonary oedema; undertransfusion means that full recovery may be delayed, and the patient may be left vulnerable to a small, additional blood loss which he could otherwise well withstand. These potential dangers may best be avoided by transfusing the patient until the c.v.p. lies at the upper limit of normal (about 12 cmH$_2$O).

(It should be noted, however, that, for reasons considered earlier, the amount of blood needed to raise c.v.p. in this way is not necessarily the amount required to restore the patient's blood volume to normal; the capacity of his circulation may be increased, e.g. by venodilatation, pharmacologically or otherwise induced.)

If, when a patient's c.v.p. has been raised to the upper limit of normal, the state of his circulation still gives cause for alarm, consideration should be given to the possibility that he is suffering from a defect of cardiac function due, for example, to cardiac tamponade, myocardial hypoxia, metabolic acidosis, etc. Further treatment should then be directed towards improving cardiac function, rather than pushing intravenous fluids to the point of causing pulmonary oedema.

Because of the sensitivity of the renal circulation to a reduction of cardiac output there is much to be said for the 'three-catheter regime', in which separate catheters are used to measure: urine flow, c.v.p. and arterial blood pressure. Of these three parameters there is little doubt that the arterial pressure is the least important.

As regards the treatment of irreversible shock (for definition see earlier), argument abounds between those who say that the correct treatment is the administration of sympathomimetic drugs to induce peripheral vasoconstriction and so increase arterial blood pressure, and those who think that tissue perfusion can best be improved by the administration of drugs, such as phenoxybenzamine, which dilate the peripheral resistance vessels and so encourage tissue perfusion, even at the expense of a further reduction of arterial pressure.

Proponents of the first line of treatment point out that the body's reaction to an acute reduction of cardiac output is sympathetically-induced vasoconstriction. They therefore argue that the administration of drugs, such as noradrenaline, which stimulate the alpha-sympathetic receptors (see section on hypertension) to cause widespread arteriolar constriction, should aid the body's physiological response to cardiovascualr stress, and should therefore help it withstand the physiological insults of the shocked state.

However, as pointed out earlier, while peripheral vasoconstriction may be beneficial in that it diverts the reduced cardiac output towards essential organs such as the brain and heart, it may also initiate ischaemic damage in the vasoconstricted tissues. The administration of alpha-stimulating sympathomimetic drugs may enhance such tissue damage, and so make the patient worse. Further, there is evidence that raising the arterial blood pressure by this means may increase the load on a heart which has been damaged by hypoxia, ischaemia, or acidosis, and may thus result in a decrease, rather than an increase, of cardiac output, and in a paradoxical worsening of the patient's condition.

The advocates for the vasodilator school of thought point out the dangers of excessive vasoconstriction as considered above, and suggest that vasodilator drugs, such as phenoxybenzamine, should alleviate sympathetically-induced tissue ischaemia, and, by lowering arterial pressure, may reduce the load on the heart, and may thus improve cardiac output and tissue perfusion. Most authorities are now moving towards this latter viewpoint. It should be pointed out, however, that sympatholytic drugs dilate all types of blood vessel, including the veins, and may therefore cause a sharp fall of c.v.p., and consequently of cardiac output. Their administration must therefore be accompanied by blood transfusion to maintain c.v.p. within normal limits, even though this may require an increase of blood volume to above the value which would be appropriate if the patient had normal sympathetic activity.

Steroids in large doses appear to cause peripheral vasodilation, rather like that induced by the alpha-blocking sympatholytic drugs; the pharmacological mechanism for this action is unknown.

If a shocked patient shows evidence of defective cardiac function, such as depressed cardiac output in the presence of a normal or high c.v.p., his clinical state may sometimes be improved by the administration of beta-stimulating sympathomimetic drugs such as isoprenaline, which increase myocardial contractility (see preceding chapter).

This treatment may be particularly effective in patients with cardiogenic shock as a result of myocardial infarction, although care must be taken that arrhythmias are promptly treated before they can cause further impairment of cardiac function.

FURTHER READING

Anon 1970 Septic shock. British Medical Journal i: 3

Barrett A M, Einstein R 1975 Catecholamines and the cardiovascular system. In: Oliver M F Modern trends in cardiology, 3rd edn. Butterworths, London, ch 2

Bloch J S, Dietzman R H, Pierce C H, Lillehei R C 1966 Theories of the production of shock. A review of their relevance to clinical practice. British Journal of Anaesthesia 38: 234

Doenicke A, Grote B, Lorenz W 1977 Blood and blood substitutes. British Journal of Anaesthesia 49: 681

Downman C B B 1972 The vasomotor centre. In: Modern trends in physiology 1. Butterworths, London

Gruber V F 1970 Recent development in the investigation and treatment of hypovolaemic shock. British Journal of Hospital Medicine 4: 631

Guyton A C 1963 Cardiac output and its regulation, 2nd edn. Saunders, Philadelphia

Hardaway R M 1968 Clinical management of shock. Charles C Thomas, Springfield, Illinois

Havard C W H 1973 Shock. In: Frontiers of medicine. Heinemann, London

Joseph S P 1976 The management of acute hypotension. British Journal of Hospital Medicine 16: 349

Kelman G R 1969 Cardiac output in shock. International Anesthesiology Clinics 7: 739

Kelman G R 1971 Interpretation of c.v.p. measurements—a review. Anaesthesia 26: 209

Kelman G R 1977 Applied cardiovascular physiology, 2nd edn. Butterworths, London, ch 4,8

Novelli G P 1975 Physiology of the shock state. In: Muchin W W, Severinghaus J W, Tiengo M, Govini S Physiological basis of anesthesiology. Pucin Medical Books

Thompson W L 1978 Drug therapy of shock. In: Turner P, Shand D G. Recent advances in clinical pharmacology. Churchill Livingstone, Edinburgh and London, ch 6

Weil M H, Shubin H 1967 Diagnosis and treatment of shock. Williams & Wilkins, Baltimore

3

Hypertension

In health, arterial blood pressure is maintained within fairly narrow limits by a variety of homeostatic mechanisms, of which the most important are the carotid and aortic baroreceptor reflexes. Some rise of arterial pressure may accompany the sympathoadrenal overactivity of exercise and emotional stimulation; but this rise is relatively small, is readily reversed, and is entirely appropriate to the body's physiological requirements of the moment. Chronic hypertension represents a very different situation: there is then a breakdown of the body's homeostatic mechanisms, allowing the arterial pressure to become chronically elevated, a condition which may have serious, and often fatal consequences on several organs, particularly the heart, brain and kidney.

Hypertension may occur in either the systemic or the pulmonary circulation. Used without qualification, however, the term usually refers to systemic hypertension.

As with many other conditions, e.g. anaemia (q.v.), it is difficult to define precisely the border-line which separates a normal blood pressure from overt hypertension. Arterial blood pressure rises slightly with increasing age, even in normal people. Moreover, in any homogeneous age group, there is a continuous gradation between the blood pressure of individuals who are clearly normal and of those who are unequivocally hypertensive. The frequency distribution curve of arterial blood pressure at any age is unimodal, therefore it is not possible to separate off a well-defined group of hypertensive patients, and to delimit these from their normal fellows.

The level of arterial blood pressure above which hypertension is considered to be present must therefore be arbitrary, but there is little doubt that, in a young adult, an arterial pressure continually above 150/95 mmHg is abnormal. Indeed, many would consider a diastolic pressure chronically in excess of this value to be an indication for treatment, even though this exposes the patient to the dangers of iatrogenic illness from therapeutical side-effects. (There is good actuarial evidence that, in any given age group, life expectancy is inversely related to the level of the diastolic blood pressure. Moreover as new drugs are developed their side effects are becoming less obtrusive; and the death rate from systemic hypertension and its complications is now falling dramatically).

Mean arterial blood pressure is, to a first approximation (see later), equal to the product of cardiac output and total peripheral resistance. Theoretically, therefore, hypertension could be due to an increase of either of these factors (or of both together). It appears, however, that systemic hypertension is usually due to arteriolar constriction, causing an increase of peripheral resistance; and, except perhaps in younger patients with labile hypertension, increases of cardiac output play little part in the pathogenesis of this condition.

It is well recognized, however, that *pulmonary* hypertension may be due either to an increase of pulmonary vascular resistance (when it is analogous to the systemic variety), or to increased blood flow through the pulmonary circulation. This latter type is found in certain forms of congenital heart disease, e.g. patent interatrial or interventricular septum or patent ductus arteriosus, in which there is left-to-right shunting of blood between the systemic and pulmonary circulations (see later).

PHYSIOLOGY

Each minute the left ventricle ejects a certain amount of blood (the cardiac output) into the aorta and its large branches. The pressure thus generated in the arterial reservoir causes blood to flow through the various body tissues in inverse proportion to their individual haemodynamic resistances. By analogy with Ohm's law (potential difference = current × resistance) it is possible to state that the pressure drop across the entire peripheral vascular bed should be approximately proportional to the product of total tissue blood flow (cardiac output) and the total resistance to blood flow (total peripheral resistance). That is:

Mean arterial pressure $\simeq$ cardiac output × total peripheral
resistance.*

This equation may be applied to either the systemic or the pulmonary circulation. Blood flow is normally the same in each case, but the haemodynamic resistance is much less in the lungs, therefore the

*This equation ignores the (normally small) pressure in the venous reservoir. Strictly, the equation should relate to arterial *minus* venous pressure, rather than to arterial pressure alone.

pulmonary arterial pressure is only about one-fifth as great as in the systemic circulation.

Peripheral resistance

The vascular bed of any given tissue may be considered to consist of a series of different types of blood vessel connected in series. Thus, in a typical tissue, the blood transverses first the arteries then, in succession, the arterioles, capillaries, venules and veins. As the arterial system branches, its total cross-sectional area increases, and at the same time the diameter of its individual vessels decreases. The former process tends to decrease the vascular resistance, the latter to increase it. But, because the resistance to blood flow provided by a given vessel is inversely proportional to the fourth power of its radius (the Hagen-Poiseuille relationship), there comes a point at which the decrease of vessel diameter becomes the dominant factor, and at this point the resistance to blood flow increases sharply.

Most of the resistance to blood flow provided by any given tissue occurs in the arterioles and precapillary sphincters which guard the entrances to the capillary bed. The major pressure drop round the circulation therefore occurs in these vessels (Fig. 3).

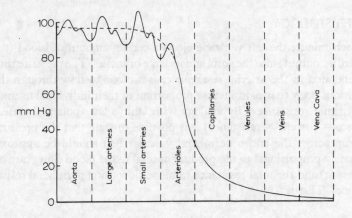

Fig. 3 Pressures in the systemic circulation (mean pressures shown by broken line).

The mean pressure in the aortic arch of a normal resting subject is approximately 95 mmHg; by the start of the arterioles this pressure has fallen by only a few mmHg, but at the arterial ends of the capillaries it has decreased to around 30 mmHg.

Changes of the resistance to tissue blood flow are brought about by changes in the tone of the smooth muscle which surrounds the arterioles and precapillary sphincters. This muscle is normally maintained in a partially contracted state by tonic sympathetic activity; and changes of vascular calibre are brought about by changes in this activity, usually reflex in response to remote stimulation.*

Changes of vascular smooth muscle tone occur also in response to changes in their chemical environment, as by local hypoxia or hypercapnia, or by circulating vasoactive hormones, such as adrenaline and noradrenaline. In the systemic circulation, hypoxia and hypercapnia cause vasodilatation: in the pulmonary circulation, hypoxia causes vasoconstriction and an increase of vascular resistance, and may thus induce pulmonary hypertension (see later).

Sympathetic adrenergic receptors in the blood vessels may be regarded as being of two types—alpha-receptors, stimulation of which results in vascular contraction, and beta-receptors, stimulation of which causes vascular relaxation. The normal postganglionic sympathetic transmitter is noradrenaline; this has chiefly alpha-adrenergic activity, therefore an increase of efferent sympathetic activity causes vasoconstriction and an increase of total peripheral resistance.

The adrenal medullae secrete both adrenaline and noradrenaline; the former stimulates predominantly beta-receptors, causing vasodilation; the latter stimulates predominantly alpha-receptors, causing vasoconstriction. An increase of adrenal medullary activity therefore results in vasodilation in those tissues, such as the skeletal muscles, which are well supplied with beta-receptors, and vasoconstriction in tissues, such as the skin, which are well supplied with alpha-receptors. Angiotensin (see below) stimulates predominantly alpha-receptors.

In addition to the state of vasoconstriction of the peripheral vessels, resistance to tissue blood flow depends on the blood viscosity. Blood which contains an excessive proportion of red cells (i.e. is polycythaemic) is unduly viscous, therefore polycythaemia tends to be associated with moderate degrees of arterial hypertension.

Autoregulation

Elementary physics predicts that blood flow through a network of rigid tubes should be directly proportional to the hydrostatic driving pressure (Fig. 4). However, blood vessels are *not* rigid tubes; and tissue blood flow is not therefore directly proportional to the difference between the arterial and venous pressures.

Firstly, an increase of intravascular pressure dilates the blood

---

*The parasympathetic division of the autonomic nervous system plays little part in the control of the peripheral resistance. With the exception of the external genitalia, the arterioles and precapillary sphincters receive no parasympathetic innervation.

vessels, causing a consequent decrease of vascular resistance. As a result, blood flow increases with an increase of intravascular pressure, even when the hydrostatic driving pressure (the difference between the arterial and venous pressures) remains constant. This fact is of considerable importance in the pulmonary circulation, where pressure

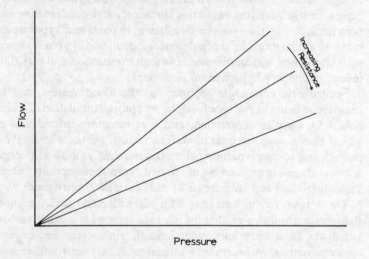

Fig. 4 Theoretical relationship between driving pressure and blood flow through a network of rigid tubes.

differences due to gravity are comparable in magnitude to the intravascular pressures, and accounts for the relative over-perfusion of the lung bases (see Chapter 4). Secondly, and more important, blood flow in many tissues is found experimentally to be relatively independent of the driving pressure; this is the phenomenon of autoregulation (Fig. 5).

There are several explanations for this phenomenon, but the most likely seems to be that a decrease of tissue blood flow, due to a decrease of arterial pressure, is accompanied by accumulation of vasodilator metabolites (carbon dioxide, ATP, lactic acid, etc.) in the vicinity of the tissue's resistance vessels; and the resulting vasodilation reduces the resistance to blood flow through the tissue until perfusion is restored almost to normal (despite the decreased arterial pressure). Conversely, an increase of arterial pressure initially causes increased tissue blood flow; this increased flow, however, rapidly washes out vasodilator metabolites, causing vasoconstriction and an increase of vascular resistance, so restoring blood flow to a level appropriate to the tissue's metabolic requirements.

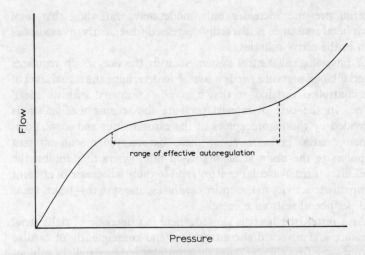

Fig. 5 Relationship between driving pressure and blood flow through an actual vascular bed—demonstrating the phenomenon of autoregulation.

The efficiency of such autoregulation varies from tissue to tissue; it is particularly in evidence in the cerebral circulation, a fact which may be related to the exquisite sensitivity of this region of the circulation to carbon dioxide.

Angiotensin
Renal ischaemia causes liberation of renin from the cells of the juxtaglomerular apparatus. This enzyme then hydrolyses a plasma α_2-globulin (angiotensinogen) into the decapeptide angiotensin I, which is then converted into angiotensin II in the plasma. This octapeptide is a very potent vasoconstrictor agent, which causes a marked increase of total peripheral resistance, both because it has a direct effect on the vascular smooth muscle and because it potentiates the noradrenaline pressor response.

Angiotensin also brings about the release of aldosterone from the adrenal cortex. This steroid sensitizes the blood vessels to the vasoconstrictor action of sympathomimetic amines; it also causes sodium retention by the kidney, thus increasing extracellular fluid volume, and possibly causing an increase of cardiac output by the Starling mechanism (see Chapter 1).

Control of arterial blood pressure
In health, arterial blood pressure is maintained within fairly narrow limits, despite wide variations of physical activity, posture, etc. During exercise there is a fivefold increase of cardiac output, yet

arterial pressure increases only moderately, indicating that total peripheral resistance is markedly decreased (due chiefly to vasodilatation in the active muscles).

A physiological control system such as the one which regulates arterial blood pressure needs a sensor to determine the actual level of the controlled variable, so that it may be compared with its 'ideal' value. In the case of arterial pressure the sensing mechanism is provided by the baroreceptors of the carotid sinus and aortic arch. When arterial pressure rises, these baroreceptors send afferent impulses to the brain at an increased rate, where they inhibit the medullary 'cardiovascular centres', and so cause a decrease of efferent sympathetic activity to the entire cardiovascular system—heart, veins and peripheral resistance vessels.

As a result, the heart is slowed, there is a decrease of right atrial pressure and myocardial contractility (and consequently of cardiac output—see first chapter), and the arterioles and precapillary sphincters are dilated, causing a decrease of peripheral resistance. There is also an increase of cardiac parasympathetic (vagal) activity, which also causes bradycardia. These changes all tend to restore arterial pressure towards normal, i.e. they form a negative feedback control system; a change in arterial pressure induces compensatory changes throughout the body in such a direction that the change of arterial pressure is minimized.

The body's compensatory responses to a fall of arterial pressure are considered further in the section on shock (q.v.).

SYSTEMIC HYPERTENSION

PATHOGENESIS

It might be thought that it would be profitable to consider the pathogenesis of hypertension in terms of factors which cause an increase of cardiac output, and factors which cause an increase of total peripheral resistance. In fact, however, it seems that all forms of sustained systemic hypertension are due to an increase of peripheral resistance, rather than to an increase of cardiac output. (The latter factor may play a part in causing the hypertension found in certain emotional states, and perhaps in causing the mild hypertension which accompanies acute expansion of the blood volume. Also, in exercise, the total peripheral resistance is reduced by vasodilatation, particularly in the active muscles, although the arterial blood pressure is moderately raised by the marked increase of cardiac output.)

It is convenient to consider first certain known causes of hyperten-

sion—renal disease, coarctation of the aorta, endocrine disease, etc.—
and then to discuss possible mechanisms for the hypertension of
unknown origin ('idiopathic' or 'essential' hypertension), which is by
far the most common type.

Renal hypertension

Bright's disease, as originally described by Richard Bright in 1827,
comprised proteinuria, a macroscopic renal abnormality and left
ventricular hypertrophy which we now know to be a result of systemic
hypertension. And it is now well recognized that renal disease and
hypertension are intimately associated: not only may primary renal
disease cause systemic hypertension, but hypertension from a non-
renal cause may, sooner or later, result in renal damage (nephrosclerosis) with aggravation of the patient's hypertensive state.

The precise pathogenesis of renal hypertension is uncertain, but the
recent development of techniques for the assay of renin and angiotensin in the plasma are rapidly improving understanding of this condition (and, indeed, of other forms of hypertension).

It is known that many forms of renal disease, ranging from
renal artery stenosis to chronic glomerulonephritis or pyelonephritis, may be accompanied by the secretion of excessive
amounts of renin from the damaged kidney(s). As renal function
deteriorates, sodium and water are retained; and consequently hypertension associated with chronic renal failure is usually due to fluid
overload. How exactly the fluid overload causes the blood pressure to
rise is not clear: in some studies it has been suggested that, initially,
there is a rise in cardiac output followed by a rise in peripheral
resistance; but the only firm fact at the present time is that the
peripheral resistance is raised in chronic renal failure. When renal
dialysis became available it was immediately clear that patients with
advanced renal failure and hypertension could be controlled by renal
dialysis alone in 90 per cent of cases. In the remaining small percentage
of patients with renal failure, the hypertension did not respond to
sodium and water removal, and has subsequently been shown to be
renin-dependent by the use of angiotensin antagonists or bilateral
nephrectomy.

Coarctation of the aorta

In this condition, the aorta is constricted at some point along its
length, commonly where it is crossed by the remains of the ductus
arteriosus. The resistance to blood flow imposed by this constriction
causes a pressure differential between the upper and lower halves of

the body; and as a result, ischaemia of the lower half can be prevented only if the pressure above the constriction is raised above normal.

Although the teleological advantages of this pressure increase are clear, the mechanism which brings it about is less so. Some workers suggest that the constriction causes a reduction of renal arterial pressure, so that the hypertension found in the upper half of the body results from renin release by the ischaemic kidneys. However, some patients are said to have a renal arterial pressure which is within, or even above, the normal range; also hypertensive patients are occasionally found with a coarctation of the descending aorta lying distal to the origin of the renal arteries.

Endocrine causes
Phaeochromocytoma

A rare, but easily understood, cause of systemic hypertension is provided by the catecholamine-secreting tumour of the adrenal medulla known as a phaeochromocytoma. Such a tumour is usually benign, and arises from chromaffin tissue rests within the adrenal gland. It secretes intermittently the vasoactive catecholamines adrenaline and noradrenaline (chiefly the latter), with the result that the patient experiences paroxysmal rises of arterial pressure, accompanied by headache, feelings of anxiety, cutaneous pallor and (often) reflex bradycardia from stimulation of the carotid and aortic baroreceptors. Ultimately, the rise of blood pressure may become continuous, a phenomenon which is also characteristic of other forms of intermittent hypertension.

Other endocrine causes

Hypertension is a feature also of various other endocrine diseases, particularly those associated with hypersecretion of adrenal cortical hormones. Thus, it occurs in Cushing's syndrome (a condition in which there is excessive adrenal cortical secretion due either to an adrenal tumour or to pituitary overactivity), and as a result of the therapeutic administration of large doses of synthetic steroids; it occurs also in primary hyperaldosteronism (Conn's syndrome).

The hypertension of these conditions appears to be due, at least in part, to the sodium retention which accompanies excessive adrenal mineralocorticoid activity. Feeding rats with large quantities of sodium chloride may induce a condition very similar to human malignant hypertension (see below), although it has been found that the administration of potassium supplements to such animals ameliorates their condition, indicating that sodium retention is not the sole etiological factor.

The mechanism by which sodium retention causes hypertension is unknown. It may act partly by increasing cardiac filling pressure, and therefore cardiac output, and partly by altering the reactivity of the peripheral resistance vessels to vasoconstrictor influences. Sodium retention is also said to cause oedema of the arteriolar walls, with a consequent increase of peripheral resistance.

Plasma renin and angiotensin levels are usually low in hypertension secondary to endocrine disease (cf. renal hypertension).

Essential hypertension

At least 90 per cent of all patients with systemic hypertension are free from any of the causes of this condition discussed above. Such patients are said to have 'idiopathic' or 'essential' hypertension.

Attempts to demonstrate a renal or endocrine basis for this condition have, in general, yielded negative results. There appears to be no abnormality of electrolyte balance; and renal blood flow and function are normal, as is cardiac output and its distribution between the various organs of the body. Some patients have increased renin and angiotensin secretion; but others, who are clinically similar, have no apparent abnormality of their renin-angiotensin system.

By definition, the etiology of essential hypertension is unknown. It is well recognized, however, that the condition is related to both genetic and environmental factors. The blood pressures of monozygotic twins are markedly similar, despite widely different environmental experiences; and there is an increased incidence of hypertension amongst the relatives of hypertensive patients. Three environmental factors have been suggested as being of particular relevance in the etiology of essential hypertension—occupational physical activity, diet (particularly sodium intake), and psychological stress—but the literature on this subject is confused, and dogmatic statements are not possible.

Whatever the primary cause of the hypertensive state, a few patients enter a so-called 'malignant phase', when the progression of their hypertension accelerates and quickly leads to death from renal failure or cerebrovascular accident (see p. 36).

Role of the renin-angiotensin system

In the majority of patients with benign (i.e. not malignant) essential hypertension, the plasma renin concentration lies within the normal range. Some patients, however, may have low plasma renin levels, even in the absence of evidence (hypokalaemia, etc.) of primary hyperaldosteronism. It appears that the renal afferent arterioles are unresponsive to stimuli which normally release renin. In patients with benign essential hypertension, plasma renin levels are negatively correlated with renal vascular resistance and glomerular filtration fraction.

In severe benign, and particularly in malignant hypertension the plasma levels of both renin and angiotensin are usually elevated, as is the rate of aldosterone secretion from the adrenal cortex.

Persistent hypertension after removal of primary cause
Certain forms of hypertension, such as that due to unilateral renal disease or a benign adrenal tumour, may be treated surgically. It is common clinical experience, however, that the blood pressure of such patients often does not return completely to normal after removal of the causative lesion. It appears that at times a raised blood pressure from whatever cause results ultimately in renal damage, so that, even after correction of the primary lesion, the patient continues to have hypertension of renal origin.

CLINICAL MANIFESTATIONS OF HYPERTENSION

In its milder forms, hypertension is symptomless, unless the patient's anxiety has been aroused by an unwise physician. More severe hypertension gives rise to headache, typically occipital and worse on awakening, dizziness or true vertigo, and impaired memory and powers of concentration. Ultimately the raised blood pressure gives rise to severe complications, affecting principally the heart, brain and kidneys.

Systemic hypertension produces left ventricular hypertrophy, which may be recognized radiographically and electro-cardiographically. Clinically, such cardiac enlargement causes a heaving apex-beat displaced downwards and outwards from its normal position (fifth intercostal space just inside the midclavicular line), accompanied by a loud first heart sound in the mitral area and a loud second sound in the aortic area. The increased strain on the left ventricle is accompanied by exertional dyspnoea, and ultimately by signs of left ventricular failure (q.v.).

The cerebral complications of hypertension include: cerebral haemorrhage, cerebral thrombosis, visual defects from hypertensive retinopathy, and hypertensive encephalopathy. In this condition the patient experiences attacks of focal cerebral ischaemia, accompanied by generalized symptoms such as fits and loss of consciousness. The pathogenesis of this potentially reversible condition is uncertain, but may include: arterial spasm, oedema of the walls of the cerebral arterioles, and the occurrence of small areas of cerebral haemorrhage or thrombosis. Malignant hypertension by definition is accompanied by renal damage and papilloedema.

Renal impairment tends to occur late, except in the malignant phase of essential hypertension, when necrotizing arteriolitis of the renal arterioles leads—in untreated patients—to a rapid impairment of renal function, and ultimately to renal failure (q.v.).

PHYSIOLOGICAL PRINCIPLES OF TREATMENT

Reduction of arterial blood pressure greatly improves the prognosis of a hypertensive patient. The therapeutic problem here is to induce an adequate reduction of arterial pressure, without, at the same time, causing too many unpleasant or dangerous side effects. An ideal antihypertensive drug would thus produce a smooth, prolonged reduction of arterial pressure, but would leave intact the normal physiological mechanisms which maintain the blood pressure in the upright position, and during exercise. Such a drug unfortunately does not as yet exist.

Until recently the corner-stone of the treatment of systemic hypertension was the use of drugs, such as reserpine, guanethidine, bethanidine, and methyl-dopa, which decrease peripheral vascular resistance, usually by an antisympathetic action. Of these drugs the only one which is still widely used is alphamethyldopa which prevents catecholamine synthesis in the sympathetic nerve terminals; and the treatment of hypertension now rests on the use of beta-blocking sympatholytic drugs, usually in combination with diuretics. By suitable regimes of these agents it is possible to reduce a patient's blood pressure to normal with a corresponding improvement in prognosis; but, despite this well-proven therapeutic efficiency, it is true to say that the mode of action of both groups of drugs is incompletely understood at the present time.

The beta-blockers—of which the most widely-used example is propranolol—decrease cardiac output, but, as explained earlier, cardiac output is not usually raised in sustained systemic hypertension, and they probably act also by reducing sympathetic activity both centrally and peripherally (perhaps thereby reducing renin release). Some workers believe that these drugs are particularly effective in patients with hypertension who have elevated plasma renin levels.

The diuretics prevent the reabsorption of sodium and water in various parts of the renal tubules (see Chapter 7), and thereby enhance sodium and water excretion. But the extracellular volume is not usually increased in ordinary hypertension, and it is therefore likely that they have an additional action on the peripheral resistance vessels.

Hydrallazine has a direct relaxing action on vascular smooth muscle. It fell out of favour some time ago because of troublesome side effects, but has recently made a comeback, and is being used increasingly—in small doses—as an adjunct to the drugs mentioned above. Sodium nitroprusside also causes dilatation of the peripheral resistance vessels, and is sometimes used to control hypertension during general anaesthesia, and to treat conditions such as hypertensive encephalopathy.

Recently drugs have been developed which block the conversion of angiotensin I to angiotensin II (see p. 31); and, although the role of angiotensin in the various forms of hypertension is still unclear, these drugs have considerable therapeutic promise.

PULMONARY HYPERTENSION

The causation and manifestations of pulmonary hypertension differ from those of the systemic variety. Pulmonary hypertension may be due either to an increase of pulmonary blood flow, or to an increase of pulmonary vascular resistance. The strain which this condition imposes affects mainly the right side of the heart, ultimately causing right ventricular failure (q.v.).

PATHOGENESIS

Increased pulmonary blood flow

At rest, cardiac output is normally of the order of 5 l/min. In patients with left-to-right shunts, however, the blood flowing through the shunt—whether through an atrial or ventricular septal defect, or through a patent ductus arteriosus—augments the right ventricular output, which thus considerably exceeds the normal 5 l/min.

This increased blood flow through the pulmonary resistance vessels causes an increase of pulmonary arterial pressure—pulmonary hypertension. Ultimately, this increased pressure causes secondary changes in the pulmonary circulation, and an increase of pulmonary vascular resistance, with aggravation of the hypertension.

In very severe cases the increase of pulmonary vascular resistance and the accompanying hypertension may be so severe that the direction of blood flow through the shunt becomes reversed, i.e. flows from right to left. This causes the patient to become desaturated. (When the condition is due to a patent ductus arteriosus, the lower half only of the body may be cyanosed, because blood to the upper half leaves the aorta above the level of origin of the ductus.)

Increased resistance to blood flow
Increased resistance to pulmonary blood flow occurs in conditions in which the systemic arterial blood gas tensions are chronically abnormal. Unlike the vessels of the systemic circulation, the pulmonary vasculature reacts to a decrease of oxygen tension by constriction and an increase of vascular resistance. Patients with chronic lung disease—particularly 'blue bloaters' (see next chapter)—may therefore have a marked increase of pulmonary vascular resistance and pulmonary hypertension. Pulmonary hypertension with right-sided heart failure from this cause is known as cor pulmonale.

In mitral stenosis, the primary haemodynamic abnormality is an increase of left atrial pressure. This increase is, however, transmitted to the pulmonary circulation because pulmonary blood flow can be maintained only when there is an appropriate pressure difference across the pulmonary vascular bed. The resultant increase of pulmonary capillary pressure tends to cause pulmonary oedema (see section on right-heart failure). In advanced cases of mitral stenosis, pulmonary arteriolar resistance increases due to medial hypertrophy, thus reducing pulmonary capillary pressure and the tendency to pulmonary oedema, but at the same time increasing the pulmonary hypertension, and strain on the right ventricle.

Obstructive pulmonary hypertension may occur also when the pulmonary vascular bed is partially occluded by multiple small pulmonary emboli. It has also been described as a result of drug toxicity, as followed the use of the anorectic drug aminorex fumarate in Europe. And 'idiopathic' cases occur sometimes in association with scleroderma or other collagen disease.

FURTHER READING

Anon 1970 Aldosterone, angiotensin and hypertension. British Medical Journal i: 769
Anon 1971 Screening for angiotensin-induced hypertension. Lancet i: 277
Anon 1971 Renal hypertension. Lancet i: 483
Anon 1976 Primary pulmonary hypertension. British Medical Journal ii: 718
Anon 1976 Hypertension—the chicken and the egg. Lancet i: 345
Anon 1979 Baroreceptors and high blood pressure. Lancet i: 1277
Anon 1979 Idiopathic aldosteronism: a diagnostic artifact? Lancet ii: 1221
Brown J J, Fraser R, Lever A F, Robertson J I S 1972 Hypertension with aldosterone excess. British Medical Journal ii: 391
Brown J J, Lever A F, Robertson J I S 1968 In: Baron D N, Compston N, Dawson A M (eds) Recent advances in medicine, 15th edn. Churchill, London
Frohlich E D 1975 Cardiovascular pathophysiology of essential hypertension. In: Zelis R (ed) The peripheral circulations. Grune and Stratton, New York, ch 12
Gabriel R 1979 Renal causes of hypertension. Practitioner 223: 211
Havard C W H 1973 Aldosterone and hyperaldosteronism. In: Frontiers of medicine. Heinemann, London

MacGregor G A 1977 High blood pressure and renal disease. British Medical Journal ii: 624

Melby L B 1968 Primary aldosteronism. Practitioner 200: 519

Peart W S 1977 The kidney as an endocrine organ. Lancet ii: 543

Pickering G 1974 Hypertension, causes, consequences and management, 2nd edn. Churchill Livingstone, Edinburgh and London

Raftery E B 1979 Hypertension—day by day. Practitioner 223: 166

Robertson D, Nies A S 1978 Antihypertensive drugs. In: Turner P, Shand D G Recent advances in clinical pharmacology. Churchill Livingstone, Edinburgh and London, ch 4

Robertson J I S 1974 Endocrine aspects of hypertension. British Journal of Hospital Medicine 11: 707

Semple P F 1979 Endocrine hypertension. Practitioner 223: 218

Swales J D 1976 The hunt for renal hypertension. Lancet i: 577

4

Respiratory failure*

The function of the lungs is to take up oxygen into the blood and to eliminate carbon dioxide from the blood; and respiratory failure occurs when they fail to perform this function adequately, i.e. when the oxygen tension (partial pressure) in the arterial blood (P_aO_2) falls below a certain level, or the arterial carbon dioxide tension (P_aCO_2) rises above a certain upper level. Obviously, the limits of P_aO_2 and P_aCO_2 outside which respiratory failure is said to exist are arbitrary; there is, however, something to be said for choosing them to coincide with levels of P_aO_2 and P_aCO_2 which have some physiological or clincial significance, such as the oxygen tension at which the steep region of the oxyhaemoglobin dissociation curve begins ($\simeq 60$ mmHg). The usual definition is that respiratory failure is present when *either* the P_aO_2 falls below 60 mmHg, (8 kPa), *or* the P_aCO_2 rises above 49 mmHg, (6.5 kPa) or both conditions occur together.

It is necessary to exclude from this definition a raised P_aCO_2 which is compensating for a metabolic alkalosis, such as may occur in pyloric stenosis accompanied by prolonged vomiting (see Chapter 12). In this situation the body is able to eliminate carbon dioxide satisfactorily, but is forced to retain it in an attempt to maintain the hydrogen ion concentration of the arterial plasma within normal limits. It is also necessary to exclude the low arterial oxygen tension which occurs in patients with congenital heart disease and anatomical right-to-left shunts; the defect here clearly lies in the heart, not in the lungs.

For reasons considered below, it is convenient to consider separetely two types of respiratory failure: type I—low P_aO_2 and a normal or low P_aCO_2; and type II—low P_aO_2 with a raised P_aCO_2.

---

*Many physiological and medical quantities are now expressed in SI units. The SI unit of pressure is the newton/m² (the pascal). Blood pressures in the wards are however still measured in mmHg, as are barometric pressures; and because arterial blood gas pressures depend crucially on the barometric pressure (especially underwater and at altitude) blood gas partial pressures in this book are still given in the units, mmHg. 1 mmHg $\simeq$ 0.13 kPa, 1 kPa $\simeq$ 7.5 mmHg.

PHYSIOLOGY

The basic function of the lungs is the exchange of oxygen and carbon dioxide through the membranes of the alveoli and pulmonary capillaries. Carbon dioxide diffuses out of the blood into the alveolar gas, oxygen diffuses in the opposite direction. The physical properties of both oxygen and carbon dioxide are such that, under almost all circumstances, there is only a very slight difference (much less than 1 mmHg) between the tensions of these gases in the alveoli and in the pulmonary end-capillary blood. Defective arterial oxygenation which was once attributed to impaired pulmonary diffusion is now thought to be due to ventilation/perfusion imbalance (see p. 44).

Pulmonary ventilation

Air is moved in and out of the lungs by the rhythmic activity of the respiratory muscles. Under normal circumstances inspiration is active, expiration is passive. When the inspiratory muscles contract they increase the volume of the thoracic cage, thus decreasing the pressure in the alveoli and causing air to enter the lungs. When the muscles relax, the elastic recoil of the lungs and chest wall causes them to return to their previous state.

The average amount of air which is moved in and out of the lungs each breath (the tidal volume) is 500 ml at rest, but considerably more during exercise. Of this volume a certain proportion—about one-third in a fit, healthy subject, but more in patients with certain forms of lung disease—is wasted in ventilating the pulmonary dead space.* This comprises the respiratory tract down as far as the respiratory bronchioles, and is the region of the lungs in which gas exchange does not occur.

Pulmonary ventilation takes place approximately 15 times each minute, therefore the amount of air which enters and leaves the pulmonary alveoli each minute (the alveolar minute volume) is approximately $\frac{2}{3} \times 0.5 \times 15 = 5$ l/min. The normal total is $0.5 \times 15 = 7\frac{1}{2}$ l/min.

When a subject is breathing a gas, such as air, which does not contain carbon dioxide, the rate of carbon dioxide elimination from the lungs equals the product of alveolar minute volume ($\dot{V}_{CO_2}$) times the fractional concentration of carbon dioxide in the alveolar gas ($F_A CO_2$). And when the body is in a steady state the rate of carbon dioxide elimination from the lungs equals the rate at which it is being produced in the tissues ($\dot{V}_{CO_2}$). If this was not the case $F_A CO_2$ would

---

*Students sometimes confuse dead space and residual volume—they are, of course, quite different.

rise or fall until alveolar CO_2 elimination *did* equal $\dot{V}CO_2$. In symbols:

$$\dot{V}_A \times F_ACO_2 = \dot{V}CO_2$$

Also, the partial pressure of carbon dioxide in the alveolar gas (P_ACO_2) is proportional to F_ACO_2, the proportionality constant being the dry barometric pressure ($\simeq 713$ mmHg at sea level). Thus, when the body is in a steady state there is the following relationship between alveolar ventilation ($\dot{V}_A$), whole body carbon dioxide production ($\dot{V}CO_2$) and P_ACO_2:

$$P_ACO_2 = 713 \times \dot{V}CO_2/\dot{V}A$$

In words, alveolar (and therefore arterial, because alveolar and arterial carbon dioxide tensions are virtually identical—see later) PCO_2 is directly proportional to the quotient of whole body carbon dioxide production divided by alveolar ventilation. *This equation is fundamental to an understanding of respiratory physiology.*

There is also a direct *experimental* relationship between alveolar (and arterial) PCO_2 and pulmonary ventilation, the latter being almost linearly related to the former (Fig. 6). Raising P_ACO_2, e.g. by rebreathing, causes an increase of alveolar ventilation to an extent that depends on the magnitude of the increase of P_ACO_2.

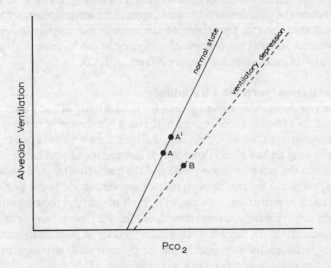

Fig. 6. Relationship between arterial PCO_2 and alveolar ventilation (for meaning of labelled points see text).

The body is normally adjusted with alveolar PCO_2 at such a level that the rate of carbon dioxide elimination by the lungs is just sufficient to eliminate its metabolically-produced carbon dioxide at the same rate as it is formed (point A, Fig. 6), and because of this relationship an increase of carbon dioxide production means that, to remain in a steady state, the body must increase either its alveolar ventilation or its alveolar PCO_2, or both. Normally both alveolar ventilation and alveolar PCO_2 increase together: the body permits its alveolar (and arterial) PCO_2 to rise until the resultant increase of alveolar ventilation is just sufficient to cope with the additional carbon dioxide load (point A', Fig. 6).

A decrease of sensitivity of the centres which control pulmonary ventilation, due for example to brain damage or chemical narcosis, means that a given level of arterial PCO_2 results in a reduced level of alveolar ventilation (broken line, Fig. 6). Ventilation therefore decreases and arterial PCO_2 rises until the body is once more in carbon dioxide balance, i.e. until alveolar carbon dioxide elimination just equals whole body carbon dioxide production. The body comes to a new equilibrium with reduced alveolar ventilation and a raised arterial PCO_2 (point B, Fig. 6). The converse obtains when the sensitivity of the respiratory centres is increased; there is then an increase of alveolar ventilation and a decrease of P_aCO_2.

Although a decrease of arterial PO_2 (arterial hypoxaemia) probably has little direct effect on the central respiratory centres, it does stimulate the peripherally-situated carotid and aortic bodies, with the result that the CO_2 sensitivity of the central receptors is indirectly increased. Arterial hypoxaemia therefore causes an increase of alveolar ventilation, accompanied by a reduction of P_aCO_2.

Ventilation/perfusion imbalance

It is physiologically advantageous for the majority of the pulmonary blood flow to go to those regions of the lung which receive the majority of alveolar ventilation. Obviously, if all ventilation went to one region of the lung and all blood flow went to another region, exchange of gas between the mixed-venous blood and the inspired air would cease. In fact, even in a normal person, pulmonary ventilation is not perfectly matched to perfusion; because, as a result of gravity, the bases of the lungs are relatively overperfused, while the apices are relatively overventilated. In disease, such inhomogeneity of pulmonary ventilation/perfusion balance may be markedly increased, although in this case the cause is not primarily gravitational.

Inhomogeneity of ventilation/perfusion balance in the lungs causes a marked decrease of arterial PO_2 and *only a very small* rise of arterial PCO_2. The reason for this important fact is discussed below.

The gas tensions in an individual alveolar-capillary unit depend on the ratio of ventilation to perfusion in that unit. Ventilation tends to raise the oxygen tension towards that of the inspired gas ($\simeq 150$ mmHg when breathing air) whereas pulmonary capillary blood flow tends to remove oxygen from the unit, thus lowering its P_{O_2} towards that of the mixed-venous blood (normally $\simeq 40$ mmHg). For the same reason, the P_{CO_2} is higher in overperfused regions of lung and lower in overventilated regions. It might be thought that, when the streams of blood from the different regions of the lung mix in the left side of the heart, the relatively well-oxygenated blood from overventilated regions would compensate for the poorly oxygenated blood from overperfused regions. This is not the case for two reasons.

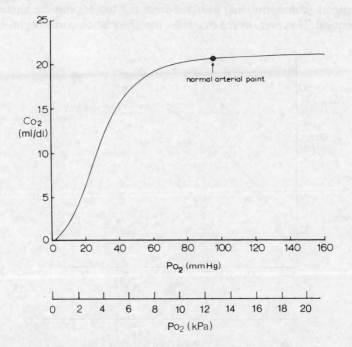

Fig. 7. Relationship between P_{O_2} and whole-blood oxygen content (P_{CO_2}). Haemoglobin concentration 15g/dl.

In the first place there is, by definition, more blood coming from overperfused regions of lung, therefore the P_{O_2} of mixed-arterial blood must be lower than the P_{O_2} of mixed-alveolar gas. (The concept of mixed-alveolar gas is a rather artificial one: it refers to the gas which would be present throughout the alveoli if their gas composition was uniform.) Similarly, the P_{CO_2} of the mixed-arterial blood tends to be higher than that of the mixed-alveolar gas, although, because of the relative shallowness of the carbon dioxide dissociation curve, the tension difference between mixed-venous blood and mixed-alveolar gas is much less in the case of carbon dioxide than in the case of oxygen, and ventilation/perfusion imbalance has only a very small effect on arterial P_{CO_2}.

In the case of oxygen there is an additional, and *more important*, reason for the fact that ventilation/perfusion imbalance lowers the P_{O_2} of the mixed-arterial blood. Although the P_{O_2} of blood from overventilated regions of lung is greater than that from regions of average ventilation/perfusion ratio, the upper part of the oxyhaemoglobin dissociation curve is almost horizontal (Fig. 7), therefore the oxygen contents (concentrations) in blood from the two regions are almost identical. However, as the P_{O_2} falls, the dissociation curve begins to

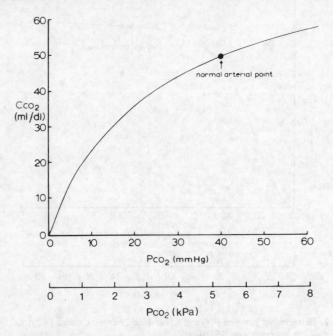

Fig. 8. Relationship between P_{CO_2} and whole-blood carbon dioxide content (C_{CO_2}). Normal metabolic (non-respiratory) acid-base state.

slope more and more steeply, so that the oxygen content of blood from relatively overperfused regions of lung (where the P_{O_2} is low) tends to be markedly reduced. When the various streams of blood mix in the left side of the heart, the relatively oxygen-deficient blood from overperfused regions pulls the mean oxygen tension down towards that of the mixed-venous blood. In contrast, the arterial P_{CO_2} is little affected by ventilation/perfusion imbalance because, over the physiological range, the relationship between blood CO_2 content and tension (Fig. 8) is almost linear (cf. the marked non-linearity of the oxyhaemoglobin dissociation curve in Fig. 7).

The alveolar air equation

Ventilation/perfusion imbalance thus causes an oxygen tension difference between the mixed-alveolar gas and the mixed-arterial blood. The magnitude of this difference provides a quantitative index of the degree of such imbalance throughout the lungs.

It is not, in practice, possible to measure the composition of the mixed-alveolar gas; instead, it is usual to calculate the composition of the so-called 'ideal alveolar gas', which has (by definition) the same P_{CO_2} as the mixed-arterial blood*, and a P_{O_2} which is calculated from a relationship known as the 'alveolar air equation'. This equation relates the oxygen tension of the ideal alveolar gas (P_{AO_2}) to the inspired oxygen tension (P_{IO_2}) and the ideal alveolar carbon dioxide tension $(P_{A CO_2} \doteq P_{a CO_2})$ as follows:

$$P_{AO_2} = P_{IO_2} - P_{ACO_2}/R$$

where R is the respiratory quotient (approximately 0.8 on a normal diet).

The substitution of representative values of P_{IO_2} (150 mmHg) and P_{ACO_2} (40 mmHg) into this equation gives a value for P_{AO_2} of approximately 100 mmHg (150—40/0.8). 100 mmHg equals 13.33 kPa. The normal arterial P_{O_2} of a fit young subject breathing air is in the region of 95 mmHg, (12.55 kPa) therefore the normal ideal alveolar-to-arterial oxygen tension difference—the (A-a) P_{O_2} difference—is approximately 5 mmHg (0.66 kPa). An increase in the value of this parameter indicates that the patient has undue ventilation/perfusion imbalance (or has a right-to-left shunt of mixed-venous blood past his lungs, a condition which may be regarded as an extreme form of ventilation/perfusion imbalance).

Respiratory acidosis**

An increase of arterial carbon dioxide tension above the normal value of 40 mmHg (5.33 kPa) is known as a respiratory acidosis (see Chapter 12). This condition is accompanied by compensatory responses which minimize the fall of plasma pH that would otherwise occur.

*Remember that ventilation/perfusion imbalance has almost no effect on the carbon dioxide tension difference between the alveolar gas and the arterial blood.

**The basic terminology of acid-base physiology is explained in Chapter 12.

Increase of plasma P_{CO_2} raises the plasma hydrogen ion concentration according to the equation:

$$CO_2 + H_2O \rightleftharpoons H^+ + HCO_3^-$$

but the increase is minimized by various buffers, of which the most important are haemoglobin and the various plasma proteins. As a result of this buffering action there is an increase of plasma bicarbonate concentration *pari passu* with the increase of P_aCO_2, and this fact may cause difficulties in the quantification of acid-base defects (see Chapter 12).

The body also reacts to a respiratory acidosis by enhanced hydrogen ion secretion into the renal tubules and retention of bicarbonate ions by the kidney. This, however, is a relatively slow process which takes several days to become completely effective. Acute carbon dioxide retention is therefore accompanied by a marked rise in plasma hydrogen ion concentration; but in chronic respiratory failure the plasma acidity may be restored almost to normal by renal compensatory mechanisms (Fig. 9). The primary respiratory acidosis (high P_{CO_2}) is then compensated by a secondary metabolic alkalosis with a high standard bicarbonate concentration (see p. 165).

PATHOPHYSIOLOGY

Type I—low P_aO_2 with a normal or low P_aCO_2

The most important cause of this type of respiratory failure is an excessive degree of ventilation/perfusion imbalance throughout the lungs, due typically to lung disease, such as bronchial asthma. This imbalance exaggerates the normal P_{O_2} difference between the alveolar gas and the arterial blood, and results in a greater or lesser degree of arterial hypoxaemia, but has little or no effect on arterial P_{CO_2}. This type of respiratory failure is sometimes seen also after trauma, particularly when this is accompanied by chest injury or fat embolism.

Arterial hypoxaemia, if sufficiently severe, stimulates the carotid and aortic chemoreceptors, and results in an increase of pulmonary ventilation with a consequent lowering of the alveolar (and therefore arterial) P_{CO_2}. This respiratory alkalosis tends to raise the alveolar oxygen tension which is determined by the alveolar air equation (see above), and thus tends to restore the arterial P_{O_2} towards normal—a compensatory mechanism which is essentially the same as that seen in subjects exposed to hypoxia on high mountains. In such conditions as chest injury, alveolar hyperventilation may also be reflexly stimulated by pulmonary congestion.

Alkalosis increases the amount of oxygen which will combine with

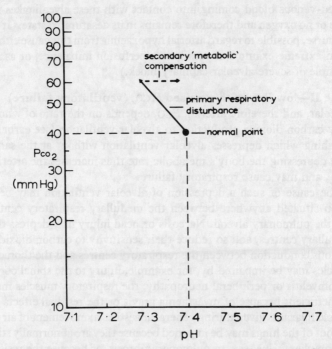

Fig. 9. Compensated and uncompensated respiratory acidosis, plotted on Siggaard-Andersen nomogram.

haemoglobin at any given oxygen tension. It therefore increases the oxygen content of the arterial blood; but, of course, it has the opposite effect in the tissues, where, by making it more difficult for the blood to give up oxygen, it tends to lower the venous oxygen tension, with possible deleterious effects on the oxygenation of cells lying near the venous ends of the capillaries.

It was formerly thought that this type of respiratory failure could result from thickening of the membrane separating the alveolar gas and the pulmonary capillary blood. It is now believed, however, that poor diffusion of oxygen is seldom, if ever, a cause of arterial hypoxaemia. The hypoxaemia which was previously attributed to 'alveolar-capillary block' is now considered to be due almost entirely to ventilation/perfusion imbalance.

In conditions such as pulmonary fat embolism, vascular channels may open up in the lungs and permit mixed-venous blood to bypass the functioning lung tissues. Such shunting of mixed-venous blood into the pulmonary veins must result in arterial hypoxaemia, and may be regarded as an extreme form of ventilation/perfusion imbalance. In pulmonary oedema alveoli may be filled with fluid, with the result that mixed-venous blood coming into contact with these alveoli takes up little or no oxygen and therefore remains in its desaturated state. (It is, of course, possible to regard arterial hypoxaemia from this cause either as an extreme example of ventilation/perfusion imbalance, or as an example of severe alveolar-capillary block.)

Type II—low P_aO_2 with a raised P_aCO_2 (ventilatory failure)

Alveolar, and therefore arterial, PCO_2 depends on the ratio of whole body carbon dioxide production to alveolar ventilation (see earlier). Anything which depresses alveolar ventilation without at the same time depressing the body's metabolic rate thus increases the arterial PCO_2, and may cause respiratory failure.

The cause of such a depression of alveolar ventilation may be a lesion situated anywhere between the medullary respiratory centre and the pulmonary alveoli. Narcosis or head injury may depress the medullary centres, and so reduce their sensitivity to carbon dioxide; nervous conduction between the respiratory centres and the thoracic muscles may be impaired by, for example, injury to the spinal cord, poliomyelitis or peripheral neuropathy; the respiratory muscles may be inefficient because of myasthenia gravis or the residual effects of muscle relaxants given during general anaesthesia; movement of air in and out of the lungs may be impeded because they are abnormally stiff (uncompliant) due, say, to pulmonary fibrosis, or because the resistance to gas flow between the atmosphere and the alveoli is increased by conditions such as laryngeal oedema, tracheal compression, or bronchiolar constriction.

An increase of alveolar PCO_2, from whatever cause, is accompanied in a patient *breathing air* by a decrease of alveolar PO_2, as predicted by the alveolar air equation (see above). This decrease of alveolar PO_2 causes a similar decrease of arterial PO_2. If the cause of the carbon dioxide retention is outwith the lungs, the alveolar-to-arterial PO_2 difference is relatively small; but if the cause of the defective alveolar ventilation is primarily in the lungs, e.g. chronic bronchitis and emphysema, there may be, in addition to alveolar hypoventilation from airway obstruction and decreased pulmonary compliance, an increase of ventilation/perfusion imbalance. Under these circumstances P_aO_2 may be disproportionately decreased, and there may be respiratory failure on both counts—$P_aO_2 < 60$ mmHg (8kPa) and $P_aCO_2 > 49$ mmHg (6.5 kPa).

CLINICAL MANIFESTATIONS OF RESPIRATORY FAILURE

Cyanosis

In theory, the clinical diagnosis of arterial hypoxaemia is straightforward, because deficient oxygenation of the arterial blood should be revealed by the patient's cyanotic colour. In practice, certain fallacies may confuse the issue.

Firstly, it is said—and it is roughly true—that cyanosis does not occur until each dl of capillary blood contains more than 5 g of reduced haemoglobin (or methaemoglobin—see below). Obviously, if the patient is anaemic, the degree of arterial hypoxaemia which is required to produce cyanosis is correspondingly increased; and if the anaemia is very severe, with a haemoglobin concentration below 5 g/dl (about 35 per cent of normal), there will be no cyanosis, no matter how severe the arterial hypoxaemia. Conversely, a patient with polycythaemia may appear cyanotic even in the absence of significant hypoxaemia.

Secondly, the presence or absence of cyanosis indicates the state of oxygenation of the blood in the capillaries of the skin or mucous membranes. This may not always indicate the state of oxygenation of the arterial blood, which is, of course, what is needed for the diagnosis of respiratory failure. If the circulation is depressed for any reason, the skin of the extremities may appear cyanotic even though there is no arterial hypoxaemia—the condition of peripheral cyanosis. For this reason, evidence of true (central) cyanosis must be sought in tissues, such as the buccal mucosa, which are always well perfused; and even here, although the colour of the mucosa correlates well with the oxygen tension of the arterial blood, the error of prediction in an individual patient is considerable.

Confusion may arise also because reduced haemoglobin is not the only pigment which can cause cyanosis. Methaemoglobin and sulphaemoglobin have absorption spectra which are similar to that of reduced haemoglobin, therefore the skin discoloration which they cause closely resembles that seen in hypoxaemia. Methaemoglobin is formed when the ferrous iron of haemoglobin is oxidized to the ferric form. Any such conversion which occurs spontaneously is normally reversed by the enzymes methaemoglobin reductase and diaphorase; absence of these enzymes causes congenital methaemoglobinaemia. Methaemoglobinaemia is caused also by oxidizing agents such as phenacetin, nitric oxide (a rare contaminant of the general anaesthetic nitrous oxide), and substituted benzene compounds such as aniline and nitrobenzene which are widely used in the chemical industry.

Hypercapnia

The clinical manifestations of hypercapnia are vague in the extreme. The patient may exhibit signs of c.n.s. depression, with drowsiness, due perhaps to carbon dioxide narcosis or to acidosis; while in severe cases he may show signs of raised intracranial pressure with headache, coma and (rarely) papilloedema. In addition, he may have evidence of a hyperdynamic circulation with warm extremities and a full, bounding pulse. Rarely there is a characteristic jerky tremor of the outstretched hands.

In practice, however, these manifestations are so non-specific that they are of little or no diagnostic value, and indeed many patients with marked carbon dioxide retention appear clinically normal.

Blood gas tensions

Because of the unreliability of the clinical signs of arterial hypoxaemia and hypercapnia, the diagnosis of respiratory failure usually rests on laboratory measurements of P_aO_2 and P_aCO_2. A sample of arterial blood can readily be obtained from the radial or brachial artery, but the accurate determination of its PO_2 or PCO_2 demands considerable care and experience.

A semiquantitative index of the state of arterial oxygenation may, however, be simply obtained by measuring the oxyhaemoglobin saturation of an arterial sample with a reflection oximeter, and then calculating its PO_2 via the oxyhaemoglobin dissociation curve. Of course, as a result of the Bohr effect, arterial oxyhaemoglobin saturation reflects both P_aO_2 and P_aCO_2, but the influence of the latter factor is not usually great. At a normal PCO_2, a PO_2 of 60 mmHg (8 kPa) corresponds to a saturation of about 90 per cent.

The extent to which a patient's respiratory acidosis is compensated or not is revealed by the nearness of the pH of his arterial blood to the normal value of 7.40. The extent of the compensation is indicated also by the standard bicarbonate concentration which is raised outside the normal range (21 to 25 mmol/1) by the compensatory metabolic alkalosis which accompanies chronic carbon dioxide retention (see Chapter 12).

Dyspnoea

Patients with various forms of respiratory failure complain of shortness of breath on quite moderate exercise, or even at rest. It is, of course, normal to become short of breath on severe exercise, but there is dispute about whether this sensation, which is familiar to us all, is the same as that experienced by patients with exertional dyspnoea brought on by lesser amounts of exercise. Campbell suggests that the sensation of dyspnoea arises primarily because there is disparity between the effort which the patient puts into his attempt to move air in and out of his lungs and the actual movement of air which he achieves.

Patients with arterial hypoxaemia may undergo anaerobic metabolism during quite mild exercise. The metabolic acidosis (see Chapter 12) thus produced (due to liberation of lactic acid from hypoxic tissues) causes a marked increase in pulmonary ventilation, and almost certainly contributes to the exertional dyspnoea which these patients experience. The exercise tolerance of such patients may, in many cases, be considerably improved by the inhalation of quite small increased concentrations of oxygen; and small, portable oxygen cylinders are now available for such use.

'Blue bloaters' and 'pink puffers'

Patients with respiratory failure due to chronic bronchitis and emphysema tend to fall into two fairly distinct categories—the 'blue bloaters' and the 'pink puffers'. The blue bloaters complain little of dyspnoea, but have marked desaturation of their arterial blood (and are therefore blue), plus right heart failure, which is responsible for their oedematous (bloated) appearance. The cause of the right heart failure (cor pulmonale) appears to be mainly an increase of pulmonary vascular resistance caused by hypoxically-induced constriction of the pulmonary arterioles—see section on pulmonary hypertension. (Unlike the vessels of the systemic circulation, the pulmonary arterioles respond to hypoxaemia by vasoconstriction, which causes an increase of pulmonary vascular resistance and pulmonary hypertension.) In contrast, the pink puffers are excessively dyspnoeic (puffing) on very mild exercise, but have little hypoxaemia, and are therefore not cyanosed (pink).

PHYSIOLOGICAL PRINCIPLES OF TREATMENT

The physiological principles of the treatment of respiratory failure are fairly strightforward. As always, however, it is necessary to remember that rules laid down by the physiologist can only be guidelines, and that, as with all clinical 'rules', exceptions abound. *Physiological dogmatism can never replace clinical experience; nor can clinical acumen compensate for a lack of physiological knowledge.*

The treatment of carbon dioxide retention is to increase alveolar ventilation. This is achieved by correction of airway obstruction, by tracheostomy and removal of bronchial secretions, and, if necessary, by artificial ventilation by mechanical means. The level of P_aCO_2 at which treatment should be instituted depends on whether the respiratory failure is acute or chronic, and on whether it is adequately compensated, i.e. on the extent to which the arterial pH departs from the normal value of 7.40. Flenley suggests that the arterial pH is a better guide to the need for treatment than the arterial PCO_2. (As always, the wisdom or otherwise of resuscitating an individual patient must be considered, and here considerable help is given by knowledge of the patient's clinical state and pulmonary function before the onset of respiratory failure.)

Lowering the patient's arterial carbon dioxide tension in this way is often sufficient to increase his P_aO_2 sufficiently to avoid hypoxia when breathing air. If this is not the case, the patient must be given additional oxygen to breathe. The hazard of giving too high an inspired oxygen concentration to a patient with chronic carbon dioxide retention, and thus depressing his alveolar ventilation by abolishing his hypoxic drive, is now well recognized* The development of apparatus, such as the Ventimask, for giving carefully controlled inspired oxygen concentrations, plus the availability of better analytical facilities for measuring P_aCO_2, make this less of a hazard than formerly.

The relief of the other type of respiratory failure, that is hypoxia without CO_2 retention, is by the administration of oxygen in a concentration sufficient to relieve hypoxaemia. Such treatment should ideally be controlled by blood-gas measurements, so that the inspired oxygen concentration can be increased until the P_aO_2 lies within the normal range. Carbon dioxide retention is not a problem in such patients, therefore giving an excessively high inspired oxygen concentration is not as dangerous as it is in patients with ventilatory failure. (It must be remembered, however, that oxygen is a drug which should be given in a carefully controlled dosage if side effects are to be avoided. The inhalation of an excessive inspired oxygen concentration for too long a period may induce signs of pulmonary oxygen toxicity, and a worsening of the patient's respiratory failure. Oxygen therapy should ideally be monitored by laboratory measurement of blood gas tensions.)

*Recent work (see Further Reading) suggests that 'hypoxic drive' in respiratory failure is dependent more on the acidity of the c.s.f. than on the PO_2 of the arterial blood.

FURTHER READING

Anon 1979 Oxygen in acute-on-chronic respiratory failure. Lancet i: 1172

Batten J C 1964 Respiratory function. In: Baron D N, Compston N, Dawson A M (ed) Recent advances in medicine, 14th edn. Churchill, London

Campbell E J M 1965 Respiratory failure. British Medical Journal i: 1451

Flenley D C 1970 Respiratory failure. Scottish Medical Journal 15: 61

Flenley D C 1978 Clinical hypoxia: causes, consequences and correction. Lancet i: 542

Havard C W H 1973 Respiratory failure. In: Frontiers of medicine. Heinemann, London

Howell J B L, Campbell E J M 1965 Breathlessness. Blackwell, Oxford

Rudolf M, Banks R A, Semple S J G 1977 Hypercapnia during oxygen therapy in acute exacerbations of chronic respiratory failure. Lancet ii: 483

Sykes M K, McNicol M W, Campbell E J M 1976 Respiratory failure, 2nd edn. Blackwell, Oxford

West J B 1970 Ventilation/blood flow and gas exchange, 2nd edn. Blackwell, Oxford

5

Anaemia

The concentration of haemoglobin in the peripheral blood of a normal adult male is in the region of 15 g/dl (15 g/100 ml), and in a normal female perhaps 2 g/dl less. Anaemia may be said to exist when this concentration falls below some arbitrary lower limit, which may perhaps be set at 13 g/dl in the male and 11 g/dl in the female.

It should be noted, however, that the peripheral haemoglobin concentration depends on both the total amount of haemoglobin present in the body and on the plasma volume. It is normally assumed (correctly) that a low peripheral haemoglobin concentration indicates a low red-cell mass; it may, however, indicate also an increased plasma volume. In pregnancy, both the plasma volume and the red-cell mass are above normal; but the increase of plasma volume is proportionally the greater, therefore the peripheral haemoglobin concentration is below normal. It is purely a matter of semantics whether this condition is classed as anaemia or not.

PHYSIOLOGY

Haemopoiesis and red cell destruction

In early embryonic life haemopoiesis is confined to the liver and spleen; but at a foetal age of about five months blood formation starts to occur also in the developing bones. After birth, haemopoiesis is confined to the bone marrow; and by the time of puberty it normally occurs only in the femoral and humeral heads, and in flat bones such as the sternum, ribs and vertebral bodies.

The stem cell which gives rise to the erythroid series of red cell precursors is probably a fixed reticuloendothelial cell. This divides to form a primitive red cell called a proerythroblast, which has basophillic cytoplasm devoid of haemoglobin. This cell then matures through the stages of early and late normoblast to become a mature erythrocyte, during which process it begins to contain haemoglobin, and its nucleus becomes pyknotic and finally disappears. The cytoplasm of the immature red cells in the peripheral blood (reticulocytes) contains RNA, which may be stained with the dye cresyl blue.

Red cell production is controlled by the hormone erythropoietin and also probably by a direct effect of hypoxia on the bone marrow. There is debate about whether the kidneys make erythropoietin as such, or whether it is formed by the action of a renal enzyme on a plasma precursor, cf. angiotensin. Patients with renal failure rapidly become anaemic (see Chapter 7), and patients with renal tumours occasionally become markedly polycythaemic.

The normal rate of red cell production is 15 to 20 ml/day; this is just balanced by red cell destruction in the liver, spleen and bone marrow. Under normal conditions, erythrocytes appear not to be destroyed until they are about 120 days old. It is thought that, initially, the cells contain enzymes which gradually become depleted as the cell ages, until finally they are unable to maintain the functional integrity of the cell membrane. When this happens the cell surface becomes altered in some way, and the cell becomes increasingly liable to phagocytosis by cells of the reticuloendothelial system.

Most of the iron which is liberated by red cell breakdown is reused, and incorporated into new erythrocytes. The remainder of the haem moiety of the haemoglobin molecule is broken down to bilirubin and excreted by the liver (see section on jaundice).

There are many different types of haemoglobin, normal and abnormal (see later); these differ in their amino acid sequences, and therefore in their oxygen carrying abilities, and other properties. In normal individuals only two types are important—haemoglobin F (Hb F) and haemoglobin A (Hb A). Throughout most of foetal life the chief oxygen carrying pigment is HbF, in which the globin part of the molecule contains two so-called α-chains and two so-called γ-chains. (These chains are characterized by the number of amino acids they contain, and their sequence). Hb F has a high oxygen affinity which helps to maintain foetal oxygenation in the relatively hypoxic intra-uterine environment. After birth Hb F is rapidly replaced by normal adult haemoglobin (Hb A), which contains two α-chains and two β-chains, and has the well-known S-shaped dissociation curve—see Figure 7. (There is also normally a small amount of Hb A_2 which has two α-chains and two δ-chains.)

Normal red cell parameters
The mature human erythrocyte is a biconcave disc with an average diameter of about 7 μm. Normally, less than 1 per cent of the peripheral red cells are reticulocytes. The number of mature red cells in the peripheral blood of the adult male is in the region of $5 \times 10^{12}/1$

(5 000 000/mm³), and in the adult female in the region of 4.5. ×
10¹²/1. The haematocrit ratio or packed cell volume is approximately
45 per cent (0.45 1/1) in the male and 40 per cent in the female.

From the red cell count (r.c.c.), the packed cell volume (p.c.v.) and
the haemoglobin concentration, it is possible to calculate other
haematological parameters, which are of help in differentiating different types of anaemia.

The mean corpuscular volume (m.c.v.) may be derived by dividing
the p.c.v. by the r.c.c., taking due care that the units are compatible.
The normal range is 78 to 94 fl*

The mean corpuscular haemoglobin concentration (m.c.h.c.) may
be derived by dividing the haemoglobin concentration by the p.c.v.
The normal range is 32 to 36 g/dl.

The mean corpuscular haemoglobin (m.c.h.) may be derived by
dividing the hemoglobin concentration by the r.c.c., again taking care
that the units are compatible. The normal range is 27 to 32 pg.

In iron deficiency anaemia there is a reduction of both m.c.v. and
m.c.h.c., i.e. the anaemia is both microcytic and hypochromic. In
anaemia from vitamin B_{12} or folic acid deficiency the m.c.v. and m.c.h.
are above normal, but the m.c.h.c. lies within the normal range. In
both cases there is a reduction of the peripheral haemoglobin concentration and r.c.c.

Requirements for normal haemopoiesis

Iron

The daily iron requirements of a normal adult male are small. Each
day, the body loses about 1 mg of iron by desquamation of cells from
the epidermis, from the gastrointestinal tract, and as red cells lost in
the urine. In females of reproductive age this iron loss is exaggerated
by the monthly loss which occurs at menstruation. This amounts to
about 1 mg of iron per day, averaged over the whole cycle, although the
menstrual loss varies widely from person to person. This iron loss
must be replaced from the diet.

Foods which are particularly rich in iron are liver, meat, peas and
eggs. An average diet contains between 10 and 20 mg of iron daily.
However, although there is apparently a safety ratio of intake over
requirement of 10:1, iron balance in the female of reproductive age is
in a precarious state, since much of the dietary iron is metabolically
unavailable. Anaemia from iron deficiency is particularly common

*Femto litre $= 1 \times 10^{-15}$ 1. The situation with regard to S.I. units in medicine is
confused at the present time. Those used in this book are mainly those adopted by the
University of Aberdeen. See also *J.clin.Path.* 1970, **23**: 818.

among working-class housewives who undergo frequent pregnancies while existing on diets which are relatively poor in iron-containing foods. (The 10 months' amenorrhoea of pregnancy results in a saving of about 200 mg of iron; but, against this, the mother has to provide iron for the growing foetus and for the blood loss which occurs at delivery. To meet these increased requirements, an average pregnancy needs about 800 mg of iron.)

Iron is absorbed mainly in the duodenum and jejunum, after being liberated from food materials by the action of gastric hydrochloric acid (see section on malabsorption syndrome). It is absorbed predominantly in the ferrous state. After absorption, it is carried in the plasma in combination with the iron-binding β-globulin, transferrin. (Ionic iron is toxic.) The normal plasma iron concentration is of the order of 100 μg/100 ml (18 μmol/1), and the plasma transferrin is normally about one-third saturated with iron.

Iron is stored within the cells of the reticuloendothelial system as the iron-containing pigments ferritin and haemosiderin. The normal adult body contains approximately 3 g of iron, of which 60 per cent is in the circulating erythrocytes, with the remainder in the myoglobin of skeletal muscles, in intracellular enzymes, and in reticuloendothelial cells in the liver, spleen and bone marrow.

Vitamin B$_{12}$ and folic acid

Normal haemopoiesis also requires adequate amounts of vitamin B$_{12}$ and folic acid. In the absence of these factors, haemopoiesis is abnormal (megaloblastic—see later), and the peripheral haemoglobin concentration is reduced.

Vitamin B$_{12}$ is found mainly in foods of animal origin, especially liver, kidney and muscle; there is very little in green vegetables, so that strict vegetarians ('vegans') may develop nutritional vitamin B$_{12}$ deficiency. The normal adult requirement is about 1 μg/day. Vitamin B$_{12}$ absorption is dependent on the presence in the intestine of a mucoprotein known as intrinsic factor. This substance is secreted by the gastric mucosa, and is therefore deficient after total gastrectomy, and when the gastric mucosa is damaged by abnormal antibodies, as in pernicious anaemia.

The most important sources of folic acid are fresh green vegetables and liver. The normal daily requirement of this vitamin is of the order of 50 μg. In contrast to vitamin B$_{12}$, folic acid is not necessary for the normal metabolism of nervous tissue; the neurological manifestations which may occur with vitamin B$_{12}$ deficiency (see later) therefore do not occur with a pure folic-acid deficiency.

ETIOLOGY

It is convenient to consider the etiology of the various forms of anaemia by dividing these into anaemias due to faulty blood formation and anaemias due to excessive loss or destruction of erythrocytes. The former may be divided into anaemias in which there is a deficiency of one or more specific chemical compounds, such as iron or vitamin B_{12}, and into aplastic anaemias, which may be 'idiopathic' or secondary to the action of drugs or other toxins. The 2nd type of anaemia may be divided into anaemias due to blood loss and anaemias due to excessive destruction of blood in the body—haemolytic anaemias.

Faulty blood formation

Bone marrow aplasia

Aplasia or hypoplasia of the bone marrow may be secondary to the toxic action of various chemicals or 'idiopathic'. In the former case the toxic action may be direct, as with antimitotic drugs, or the result of an individual idiosyncrasy to a certain drug. Drugs which commonly cause aplastic anaemia include chloramphenicol, phenylbutazone, gold compounds used in the treatment of rheumatoid arthritis, and thiouracil. Marrow hypoplasia may occur also as a result of the action of ionizing radiations. Benzene used to cause aplastic anaemia in industry, but is now little used. 'Toxic anaemia' in industry is notifiable under the Factories Act of 1961.

In most cases the peripheral blood cells are normochromic and normocytic, with hypoplasia of the bone marrow. There may also be a haemolytic element with shortening of red cell survival time. Aplastic anaemia is usually accompanied by defective production of all the formed elements of the blood (pancytopenia). There may thus be an increased liability to infection, and an accompanying haemorrhagic tendency from platelet deficiency (thrombocytopenia—q.v.), so that the anaemia is aggravated by the effects of chronic haemorrhage.

Iron deficiency

Iron deficiency is by far the commonest cause of anaemia. Even on a good diet, iron balance is precarious in the normal female of reproductive age (see above), and even a slight, additional demand, e.g. due to menorrhagia or frequent pregnancy, may be sufficient to cause a negative iron balance. In both sexes iron deficiency may occur as a result of chronic haemorrhage (see below) or intestinal malabsorption (q.v.). Iron deficiency is especially likely in Asian immigrants to this country because their diet contains relatively large amounts of phosphates and phytic acid which impede iron absorption. In infants, iron deficiency occurs if milk feeding is unduly prolonged, because milk is relatively poor in iron. This danger is particularly severe in premature babies, who are born without the normal iron reserves which are laid down in late pregnancy.

Negative iron balance depletes first the body's iron stores, and then causes a fall of the plasma iron concentration (normally 60 to 150 μg/100 ml, but with a considerable diurnal swing) and desaturation of the iron-combining protein, transferrin (normally about 30 per cent saturated). When the transferrin saturation falls to about one-half its normal value, the peripheral blood begins to show the typical picture of a microcytic, hypochromic anaemia, with an m.c.h.c. of less than 30 g/dl. There may also be additional non-haematological signs of iron deficiency, such as koilonychia, chronic atrophic glossitis and angular stomatitis, which may be due to deficiency of various (unspecified) iron-containing intracellular enzymes.

Vitamin B_{12} and folic acid deficiency

Deficiency of vitamin B_{12} and folic acid gives rise to an anaemia which is characterized by the presence, in the bone marrow, of abnormal cells called megaloblasts. These are somewhat larger than the normal red cell precursors (normoblasts), and have nuclear chromatin which is more loosely woven. Such megaloblastic anaemias are characterized by defective nucleoprotein synthesis, not only in the red cell precursors, but also in the precursors of other blood cells, and in endothelium generally, with the result that the patient may have symptoms such as anorexia and diarrhoea, which are not due primarily to his reduced peripheral haemoglobin concentration.

Megaloblastic blood formation is accompanied by the presence of abnormal erythrocytes in the peripheral blood. These cells may be of strange shapes (poikilocytosis), and lack the uniformity of size which characterizes the normal peripheral blood picture (anisocytosis). In addition, the cells are larger than normal (macrocytic—m.c.v. > 94 fl), and contain a greater than normal amount of haemoglobin (m.c.h. > 32 pg). The intracellular haemoglobin concentration is, however, normal (approximately 35 g/dl).

(It should be noted that a macrocytic peripheral blood picture is not necessarily the result of megaloblastic haemopoiesis; it occurs, for example, also in certain haemolytic states, aplastic anaemia, etc.)

Vitamin B_{12}

Dietary vitamin B_{12} combines with intrinsic factor in the stomach, and is absorbed from the terminal ileum. Dietary deficiency of this vitamin is rare, except in the tropics, when it is accompanied by multiple vitamin and other deficiencies, as in tropical malnutrition (kwashior-kor). It occurs also in total vegetarians.

Lack of intrinsic factor causes vitamin B_{12} deficiency, and arises either as a result of Addisonian pernicious anaemia, when the gastric mucosa is damaged, probably by an autoimmune process, or as a result of total (or, rarely, partial) gastrectomy. After total gastrectomy the body's stores of B_{12} are sufficient to last for several years; overt signs of deficiency from this cause are therefore rare, because total gastrec-tomy is usually performed for gastric carcinoma, the prognosis of which is notoriously bad. Deficiency of vitamin B_{12} may also be a feature of the malabsorption syndrome (q.v.).

The diagnosis of vitamin B_{12} deficiency may be made by estimation of its concentration in the peripheral blood; the lower limit of normal is around 150 ng/1. Deficiency may also be detected by the Schilling test, in which the patient is given orally a dose of radioactive B_{12}, followed by a large injection of non-radioactive vitamin. This second dose greatly increases the rate of B_{12} excretion, with the result that, if it has been absorbed, the radioactive vitamin is excreted by the kidneys and may be measured in the urine. In a normal person more than 15 per cent of the orally administered (radioactive) vitamin may be recovered in this way.

In addition to the usual non-specific manifestations of anaemia (see later), patients with pernicious anaemia may have a variety of non-haematological manifestations of vitamin B_{12} deficiency, including glossitis, gastrointestinal disturbances, and neurological abnormalities such as paraesthesiae, impaired cutaneous sensation and muscular weakness. There may also be signs of subacute combined degeneration of the posterior and lateral columns of the spinal cord, with impaired vibration and position sense, and extensor plantar responses. In addition, the patient may show psychiatric abnormalities, such as depression and irritability.

Folic acid

As is the case with vitamin B_{12}, obvious dietary deficiency of folic acid is rare, although a suboptimal intake may, in fact, be quite common. Deficiency occurs in the malabsorption syndrome (q.v.), and in any condition in which there is rapid cell synthesis. Thus, folate deficiency may occur in haemolytic anaemia, in leukaemia and in patients with carcinomatosis. It may occur also in pregnancy, when absorption has to keep pace with the needs of the growing foetus. Folate deficiency is found in patients who are taking certain anticonvulsant drugs, such as phenytoin and phenobarbitone; it appears that these drugs compete for metabolic pathways which normally utilize folic acid. Deficiency may occur also in patients who are being treated for neoplastic blood disorders with folic acid antagonists, such as methotrexate.

The biochemical confirmation of folate deficiency is unreliable; and, in practice, the diagnosis is usually made by the finding of a megaloblastic anaemia in the absence of vitamin B_{12} deficiency. The plasma folate level in this condition is usually below 3 $\mu g/l$.

Excessive blood loss or destruction

Haemorrhage

Chronic haemorrhage gives rise to iron deficiency anaemia (see above). Acute haemorrhage, however, does not immediately produce anaemia in the sense of a reduction of the peripheral haemoglobin concentration, although, of course, it reduces the total red-cell mass. In fact, the requirement of a patient soon after an acute haemorrhage is not so much for haemoglobin as for an adequate circulating blood volume (see section on shock). The body is far less tolerant of a reduced circulating blood volume than of a low haemoglobin concentration; and it is common practice to treat acute haemorrhage by the transfusion of non-haemoglobin containing fluids, with the result that the circulating blood volume is restored to normal, while the peripheral haemoglobin concentration is reduced in proportion to the original blood loss. (Such treatment is, of course, only speeding up the body's normal defence mechanism against acute hypovolaemia, i.e. the transfer of interstitial fluid into the intravascular compartment.)

The anaemia which occurs some hours after an acute haemorrhage is normocytic and normochromic. However, if the body's iron reserves are insufficient to allow it to make good the red cell loss the typical microcytic, hypochromic anaemia of chronic iron deficiency gradually develops.

Haemolytic anaemias

Anaemia occurs when red cells are lost from the body or destroyed faster than they can be replaced by the bone marrow. Thus anaemia occurs when erythrocytes are destroyed at an abnormal rate, so that haemopoiesis is unable to keep pace with the increased cell destruction. If the increased red cell destruction is adequately compensated by increased marrow activity, the patient may not be anaemic, although he will show manifestations of increased haemolysis — haemolytic jaundice, q.v. Normal marrow is able to compensate for a reduction of red cell survival time down to about 20 days. In severe cases, however, red cell survival may be reduced to as short as five days, and, under these circumstances, severe anaemia is inevitable.

Haemolytic anaemia may arise from the action of certain drugs and other toxins, as a result of congenital abnormalities of the red cells, or as a result of abnormal antibodies in the circulating blood.

Haemolysis caused by drugs

The haemolytic action of some drugs is due to a direct toxic action on the erythrocytes. The phenomenon is then dose-dependent, although the sensitivity of different individuals varies somewhat, presumably as a result of constitutional factors. This type of haemolysis occurs with many drugs, including phenylhydrazine, arsenic and sulphonamides, and with bacterial toxins.

The other type of drug-induced haemolysis occurs with relatively small doses of certain drugs, but in only a small proportion of the patients at risk, i.e. it is a form of 'sensitivity reaction'. It is now known that many of the patients affected by this type of haemolysis have red cells which are deficient in the enzyme glucose-6-phosphate dehydrogenase (G-6-PD). G-6-PD deficiency is a sex-linked, inherited defect of intermediate dominance, and is particularly common in American Negroes, 10 per cent of whom are affected.

In patients with G-6-PD deficiency the red cells are deficient in the enzyme which is normally responsible for maintaining cellular glutathione in the reduced form, as it must be if it is to prevent cellular damage. In the absence of reduced glutathione, oxidizing agents denature the intracellular proteins and the globin moiety of the haemoglobin molecule, with the result that the cells are damaged and thus become haemolysed. In some cells the denatured haemoglobin precipitates out in the cytoplasm as 'Heinz bodies'.

Many drugs will cause haemolysis in patients with G-6-PD deficiency, including antimalarials (which were the first drugs to be incriminated in this condition), nitrofurantoin, and sulphonamides. In addition, severe haemolysis may follow the ingestion of partially-cooked broad beans (*Vicia faba*)—the condition of favism.

Hereditary spherocytosis

Hereditary spherocytosis is inherited as a Mendelian dominant, and is characterized by the presence in the peripheral blood of erythrocytes which are both of smaller diameter than normal, and, at the same time, more spherical ('microspherocytes'). The fundamental defect in this condition seems to be abnormal permeability of the cell membrane to sodium ions, with the result that the cells become swollen by excess intracellular fluid and electrolytes. These microspherocytes are abnormally fragile when exposed to hypotonic saline—a fact of diagnostic importance. They are also particularly liable to sequestration in the spleen, with the result that the mean red cell survival time is reduced, and the patient shows evidence of increased haemolysis. Splenectomy results in the clinical cure of almost all patients, although it has little effect on their basic red cell abnormality.

Hereditary non-spherocytic haemolytic anaemia and congenital elliptocytosis are much rarer causes of haemolytic anaemia, in which splenectomy results in cure much less certainly.

The haemoglobinopathies

There is also a large group of patients with haemolytic anaemia in which the primary defect is in haemoglobin synthesis. The most important of these conditions are thalassaemia (Mediterranean anaemia) and sickle cell disease. Thalassaemia is especially common in S E Asia, and in people who live around the Mediterranean.

In thalassaemia the primary defect is a genetically-determined quantitative defect of haemoglobin synthesis, affecting the globin moiety of the molecule. The defect can involve either the α-chains, leading to α-thalassaemia, or the β-chains, leading to β-thalassaemia. The condition may be either heterozygous (thalassaemia minor) or homozygous (thalassaemia major). The homozygous form of α-thalassaemia is lethal *in utero*, causing hydrops foetalis.

Thalassaemia minor is a relatively benign condition, and many patients with this disorder are symptom-free. Thalassaemia major is a serious illness, starting in infancy and manifested by severe anaemia and evidence of haemolysis, with splenomegaly, an increased peripheral reticulocyte count, mild jaundice and increased faecal bilirubin excretion. As in other forms of haemolytic anaemia, there may be chronic ulceration of the legs.

Although the patient may be severely anaemic there is no evidence of iron deficiency; the serum iron concentration is normal or raised, and the iron-binding protein transferrin is normally saturated.

The other condition in which an abnormality of haemoglobin synthesis is accompanied by excessive haemolysis is sickle cell disease. In this condition the red cells contain an abnormal form of haemoglobin—Hb S—with abnormal β-chains. As a result of this abnormality, they take on bizarre shapes ('sickling') when their environmental oxygen tension is reduced below a certain critical level. This change of shape is due to a physiochemical change in the haemoglobin molecule, and (as in spherocytosis) it renders the cell abnormally liable to destruction in the spleen. Sickle cell disease becomes apparent only after birth, when the foetal haemoglobin (α and γ-chains) of the newborn infant becomes replaced by (abnormal) adult haemoglobin (α and β-chains). The disease may exist in either the homozygous or the heterozygous form (sickle cell trait).

The condition is interesting in that possession of the sickle cell trait protects against falciparum malaria; it is therefore very common amongst Negroes; and in American blacks the incidence is about 10 per cent. The other haemoglobinopathies may also have a similar survival value, a fact which explains why they have not 'died out' during the course of evolution.

Autoimmune haemolytic anaemia

The last important cause of excessive haemolysis is the presence, in the plasma, of abnormal antibodies to the patient's own red cells. Such antibodies may be either 'warm' (active at 37°C) or 'cold' (active at lower temperatures). In the former case the antibody is a low molecular weight globulin (IgG); in the latter case it is a globulin of higher molecular weight (IgM). In both cases the antibody becomes attached to the red cell membrane, where its presence may be demonstrated by the direct Coombs' test, in which antibodies, prepared against human globulin, cause agglutination of the patient's affected red cells.

Autoimmune haemolytic anaemia may occur in the course of some other disease, such as chronic lymphatic leukaemia or reticulum cell sarcoma, or it may be 'idiopathic'. It is not known whether the primary abnormality is a change in the antigenicity of the patient's red cells, or in his antibody-producing tissues. The condition may be of all grades of severity, from an acute, febrile illness, in which red cell destruction is so rapid that haemoglobin appears in the urine, to a mild and well compensated haemolytic jaundice.

Pneumonia from infection with *Mycoplasma pneumoniae* may be . followed several weeks later by a cold antibody haemolytic anaemia; this condition may be wrongly attributed to sulphonamide toxicity.

CLINICAL MANIFESTATIONS OF ANAEMIA

The clinical manifestations of anaemia are relatively non-specific, and correlate badly with its severity, as assessed by reduction of the peripheral haemoglobin concentration. The most important physical sign of anaemia is obviously pallor, particularly of the mucous membranes; but the false diagnosis of anaemia on the basis of fancied pallor is too common an occurrence to need detailed comment here, except to reiterate that the diagnosis can be made with certainty only on the basis of a measured haemoglobin concentration which is significantly below normal.

In anaemia, the oxygen-carrying power of the blood is reduced, (Fig. 10, cf. Fig. 7); therefore, if the supply of oxygen to the tissues is not to be jeopardized, the heart has to pump blood round the body at an increased rate. Anaemic patients thus show signs of increased cardiac activity, with tachycardia and palpitations. They may also have so-called 'haemic' murmurs, caused by the fact that blood-flow through the cardiac valves is turbulent where it would normally be streamline—a transition which depends partly on the increased flow velocity and partly on reduced blood viscosity.

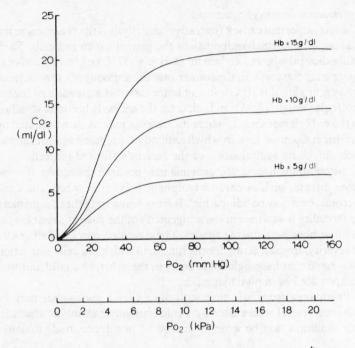

Fig. 10. Relationship between P_{O_2} and whole blood oxygen content (C_{O_2}) for bloods of different haemoglobin concentrations.

Poor blood supply to the peripheral tissues gives rise to various non-specific manifestations, very like those of chronic heart failure (q.v.). Thus there may be easy fatigability of skeletal muscles, paraesthesiae from poor oxygenation of peripheral nerves, lethargy from cerebral hypoxia, and anorexia and flatulence as a result of poor oxygen supply to the gastrointestinal tract. Dyspnoea tends to occur on quite moderate exertion, because the blood flow to the skeletal muscles cannot increase sufficiently to prevent anaerobic metabolism, even at relatively light work loads.

The increased strain on the heart may ultimately cause heart failure (q.v.). This tendency is aggravated by the fact that the myocardium is required to perform extra work at a time when its oxygen supply is inadequate, because of the reduced peripheral haemoglobin concentration. For the same reason, angina is common.

Iron deficiency anaemia may be accompanied by koilonychia, glossitis and angular stomatitis, and by dysphagia from the oesophageal web of the Plummer-Vinson syndrome. Anaemia from vitamin B_{12} deficiency may be accompanied by the manifestations of peripheral neuropathy, and by subacute combined degeneration of the spinal cord, in which there is progressive degeneration of the posterior and lateral columns, causing disturbances of sensation and, less commonly, signs of upper motor neurone paresis.

FURTHER READING

Anon 1971 Iron. Lancet ii: 475
Anon 1977 Erythropoietin. Lancet i: 1137
Anon 1978 Fetal haemoglobin in sickle-cell anaemia and thalassaemia—a clue to therapy. Lancet i: 971
Anon 1979 Serum-ferritin. Lancet i: 533
Bartos H R, Desforges J F 1967 Drug-induced blood dyscrasias. Practitioner 199: 37
Blackburn E K 1967 The megaloblastic anaemias. Practitioner 199: 14
British Medical Bulletin 1976 Haemoglobin: structure, function and synthesis. 32: 193
Campbell E J M, Dickinson C J, Slater J D H 1974 Clinical physiology, 4th edn. Blackwell, Oxford, ch 6
Cumming R L C 1978 Disorders of iron metabolism. Practitioner 221: 184
Dacie J V 1962 Haemolytic mechanisms in health and disease. British Medical Journal ii: 429
Dacie J V 1970 Autoimmune haemolytic anaemias. British Medical Journal ii: 381
Dawson A A, Walker W 1974 Blood formation and the pathogenesis of anaemia. British Medical Journal ii: 260
Huehns E R 1967 Thalassaemia. Practitioner 199: 51
MacIver J E 1976 Haematological problems in immigrants. Practitioner 261: 50
Maclean N 1978 Haemoglobin. Edward Arnold, London
Marengo-Rowe A J 1971 Haemoglobinopathies. British Journal of Hospital Medicine 6: 617
Peart W S 1977 The kidney as an endocrine organ. Lancet ii: 543
Prankerd T A J 1975 The assessment of bone marrow function. British Journal of Hospital Medicine 14: 259
Thompson R B 1979 A short textbook of haematology, 5th edn. Pitman, London
Weatherall D J 1978 Haemolytic anaemia. Practitioner 221: 194

6

Haemorrhagic disorders

The body possesses several mechanisms for minimizing blood loss following all but major trauma, and impairment of any one of these mechanisms causes a haemorrhagic state, which may be manifest either as prolonged bleeding after minor trauma or as spontaneous haemorrhage from mucous membranes, and into the skin, joints and internal organs.

A major part of the body's defence against haemorrhage is the complex series of enzymatic processes by which the soluble protein, fibrinogen, is converted into insoluble fibrin. This fibrin then forms a plug, which occludes the damaged vessels and prevents further blood loss. The complex process which is responsible for converting fibrinogen into fibrin may be deranged by deficiency of one or more essential clotting factors, as in the genetically determined conditions, haemophilia and Christmas disease, and the acquired condition of hypoprothrombinaemia, which may accompany vitamin K deficiency or hepatic disease (q.v.).

The body possesses also a mechanism for the prevention of spontaneous intravascular thrombosis. This mechanism may, however be overwhelmed when large amounts of thromboplastin (probably factor III—see later) enter the circulation, for example as a result of concealed retroplacental haemorrhage. There is then extensive intravascular conversion of fibrinogen into fibrin, with a resulting deficiency of fibrinogen and other clotting factors, and a consequent haemorrhagic tendency (the acute defibrination syndrome or disseminated intravascular coagulation).

A bleeding tendency may arise also as a result of a defect in the body's other antihaemorrhage mechanisms. These consist of the localized vasoconstriction of damaged blood vessels and the plugging of defects in the vascular endothelium with platelet aggregates.

PHYSIOLOGY

There appear to be three basic mechanisms which are concerned with the control of bleeding following local trauma—constriction of the injured vessels, aggregation of platelets at the site of injury, and formation of a fibrin clot. The first two processes reduce the rate of blood flow through the injured vessel, and thus aid fibrin deposition and efficient haemostasis. In the absence of such preparatory slowing, fibrin is deposited as long ribbons, rather than as a solid plug, and the efficiency of haemostasis is consequently impaired.

Contraction of vascular smooth muscle

The role of vasoconstriction in the control of haemorrhage is not completely clear. It is known that the traumatic avulsion of a limb may be followed by such intense vascular spasm that little blood loss occurs; but, on the other hand, with a clean surgical incision this mechanism is far less efficient, and severe haemorrhage may occur unless the damaged vessels are mechanically occluded.

In the nail-beds, the capillary loops may be observed under a dissecting microscope, and can be seen to become obliterated in response to local trauma—a response which depends on constriction of arterioles and precapillary sphincters, because the capillaries have no power of independent contraction. But in other regions of the body there is evidence that the microcirculatory response to injury is much less marked. Von Willebrand's disease was formerly cited as an example of a haemorrhagic tendency from defective vascular contractility; but it is now known that this condition is associated also with deficiency of certain clotting factors, chiefly factor VIII (see later), and this deficiency is now thought to be the main etiological factor.

Platelets

The platelets are anuclear cells approximately 2 μm in diameter; they are formed in the bone marrow from megakaryocytes. The normal platelet count in the peripheral blood is of the order of $250 \times 10^9/1$.

Platelets are essential both for the control of bleeding following trauma, and for maintenance of the normal integrity of the vascular endothelium. Platelet deficiency (thrombocytopenia) results in excessive bleeding after trauma and in spontaneous bleeding into the skin and from mucous membranes (purpura). The platelets are normally concentrated in the peripheral layers of the flowing blood; and it is thought that from there they are continually deposited onto the vascular endothelium, where, in some unknown way, they help to maintain its functional integrity.

The platelets are concerned with the control of traumatically-induced haemorrhage. They congregate around the site of a breach in the vascular endothelium, and, in this way, can seal a vessel up to the size of an arteriole. They also release a factor—perhaps 5-hydroxy-tryptamine (5-HT)—which causes or accentuates the vasoconstriction mentioned earlier. In larger vessels, platelet thrombi partially occlude the vascular lumen at the site of injury, and thus aid efficient fibrin deposition.

Platelet aggregation around a vascular injury involves at least two mechanisms: platelets adhere to exposed collagen fibres; they also tend to aggregate in the presence of adenosine diphosphate (ADP), which is released from ruptured platelets. Platelets rupture on contact with foreign surfaces, i.e. with any surface which is not normal vascular endothelium.

Platelets are concerned also with the clotting process (see below); on contact with a foreign surface they release a phospholipid which is involved in several stages of the clotting process.

Blood coagulation

Blood coagulation is an extremely complex process, the final step of which involves the conversion of fibrinogen into fibrin by the proteolytic enzyme, thrombin. The fibrin filaments so formed entrap erythrocytes and other formed elements of the blood to produce a firm clot, which occludes the damaged vessel and prevents further haemorrhage.

At least twelve different plasma components are concerned in the clotting process (Fig. 11). These factors have been given the Roman numerals from I to XIII, roughly in the order in which they were discovered. Thus, thrombin is now known as factor II, fibrin as factor I, and antihaemophilic globulin as factor VIII. Most of these factors are proteins which are synthesized in the liver.

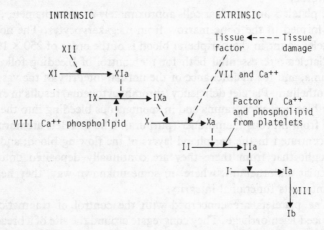

Fig. 11. Current hypothesis of blood coagulation (after Macfarlane, 1964)

The general pattern of blood coagulation is that one factor is converted enzymatically into its active form, which can then activate a factor further along the chain. (It is now known, however, that the original system proposed by Macfarlane is an over-simplification, and that complex biochemical feedback pathways exist between the various factors.) At each stage the number of molecules involved is multiplied at least ten times; at the same time, the speed of the conversion process is greatly enhanced. Thus, the activation of a relatively few molecules of one of the early factors can result in the final formation of millions of molecules of fibrin, and in the formation of a large clot.

There are two basic divisions of the clotting mechanism—intrinsic and extrinsic. The final steps after the activation of factor X are, however, the same in each case.

The intrinsic mechanism involves factors which are found solely in the plasma. It is initiated by the conversion of factor XII into its active form, factor XIIa, a process which involves the plasma polypeptide kallikrein. The activated factor XII then activates successively factors XI, IX, X and II, until finally fibrinogen is split into fibrin. Factor XIII is necessary to polymerize the newly formed fibrin (factor Ia) into a stable clot (factor Ib); active factor XIII is formed from its inactive precursor by the action of thrombin in the presence of calcium ions. In addition, thrombin accelerates activation of several of the earlier factors involved in the intrinsic clotting system, and enhances liberation of ADP from platelets (see earlier).

The extrinsic clotting mechanism involves the liberation from damaged tissues of a substance (factor III) which, in the presence of factor VII, activates factor X, and thus bypasses several of the earlier, and slower steps of the intrinsic system.

Calcium ions (factor IV) are involved at several points in both the intrinsic and extrinsic clotting processes.

Full understanding of the normal clotting mechanism presents a considerable intellectual challenge; but an equally important question is: what normally prevents coagulation intravascularly? Random processes might be expected to initiate the activation of a small quantity of factor XII, and this, by the amplification system mentioned above, would be expected to activate progressively increasing amounts of intermediate factors, until finally a large fibrin clot would be formed. Yet intravascular clotting does not normally occur. Why not?

It appears that, under normal circumstances, a small quantity of fibrin does indeed become formed intravascularly, where it tends to deposit onto the vascular endothelium. This fibrin is, however, normally removed, as rapidly as it is formed, by the action of circulating fibrinolytic enzymes (plasmins or fibrinolysins). These enzymes are formed by the activation of inactive plasminogen precursors. Appropriate activators are found in vascular endothelial cells, and in the urine where they may be concerned with maintaining the patency of the uriniferous tubules. (Plasma contains also a plasmin antagonist which is able to prevent the development of excessive fibrinolytic activity in the blood.) In addition, plasma may contain a thrombin inactivator, which helps to prevent intravascular coagulation. Also, the cells of the reticuloendothelial system may be able to remove small quantities of activated clotting factors from the plasma, should these appear.

Despite recent advances in our knowledge of fibrinolytic mechanisms, our understanding of how the body achieves a balance between fibrin deposition and fibrinolysis is far from complete. Such understanding is of course of considerable importance because of the possibility of therapeutic intervention in thrombotic situations by means of plasmin activators such as streptokinase (see Further Reading).

Tests of haemostatic ability

Clotting time
The whole blood clotting time is simply a measure of the ability of the patient's blood to clot *in vitro*, either at 37°C or at room temperature. The upper limit of normal is roughly 10 minutes; but it may be considerably prolonged in haemophilia (q.v.), and similar disorders. This test is now seldom used clinically.

Bleeding time
This test measures the ability of injured small blood vessels to contract, and the ability of platelets to aggregate and plug a vascular defect. The details of the technique vary from centre to centre: in principle however a small prick is made in the ear-lobe to a depth of a few mm and the time taken for blood flow to stop. Blood which oozes from the wound must be removed with filter paper every 30 seconds to prevent haemostasis from the normal clotting mechanism. The bleeding time may be prolonged in thrombocytopenia (q.v.), and with vascular defects e.g. scurvy.

Capillary fragility test (Hess' test)
In this test a blood pressure cuff is applied to the upper arm, and maintained at a pressure midway between systolic and diastolic for 5

minutes. In patients with vascular defects, or quantitative or qualitative platelet deficiencies appreciable numbers of punctate haemorrhages (petechiae) appear below the cuff.

In practice none of the above tests is very precise, but in recent years biochemical tests have become available which, although complicated in themselves, greatly simplify diagnosis of the haemorrhagic disorders. Only a very brief outline of this complex subject will be given here.

One-stage prothrombin time
Tissue extract and calcium are added to a sample of the patient's plasma (which has previously been rendered incoagulable by the removal of calcium ions with oxalate, citrate or 'Sequestrene'), and the time for a clot to form is measured. This test is abnormal when there is a deficiency of prothrombin, fibrinogen, or of factors V, VII or X. It is used for the control of anticoagulant therapy.

Thromboplastin generation test
In this test the patient's plasma is separated into several fractions, each one of which contains only some of his various clotting factors e.g. only factors V and VIII. The missing factors are then added, and the amount of 'thromboplastin'* generated in a given time is assayed by measuring its ability to convert normal fibrinogen into fibrin. In this way it is possible to define fairly precisely which factor(s) are missing from the patient's blood.

HAEMORRHAGIC DISEASES

A haemorrhagic tendency may manifest itself either as excessive and/or prolonged bleeding from relatively minor trauma, or as spontaneous haemorrhage into the skin or internal organs. Such a pathological state may result from a deficiency of one or more of the normal plasma clotting factors, from a qualitative or quantitative abnormality of the platelets, and from an abnormality of the blood vessels themselves.

Deficiency of plasma clotting factors
A haemorrhagic tendency from this cause may arise either as a genetically-determined deficiency of a single factor, e.g. haemophilia (factor VIII) or Christmas disease (factor IX); or it may be the result of

*Activated factor X reacts with factor V, phospholipid and calcium to form an enzyme which converts prothrombin into thrombin. This complex is known as thromboplastin.

impaired synthesis of several clotting factors, as in hepatic disease, vitamin K deficiency, or after the administration of vitamin K antagonists, such as the coumarin anticoagulants.

Genetically-determined deficiencies of most of the individual plasma clotting factors have been described, but, with the exception of haemophilia and Christmas disease, such deficiencies are excessively rare.

Vitamin K deficiency

Vitamin K is a fat-soluble vitamin, deficiency of which produces a lack of several hepatically-produced clotting factors. Factor VII is the first to be affected, followed by factors II, IX, and X. This condition occurs when vitamin K absorption is impaired by biliary obstruction or the malabsorption syndrome (q.v.), or in haemorrhagic disease of the newborn, when the deficiency arises partly from metabolic immaturity of the neonatal liver and partly from the fact that the intestinal bacteria, which normally synthesize a proportion of the body's vitamin K, have yet to become established. A rather similar situation occurs when the liver's synthetic ability is impaired by disease (see Chapter 8), or by the administration of coumarin anticoagulants.

Haemophilia

Haemophilia is a recessive, sex-linked, genetically-determined condition in which there is deficiency of factor VIII (antihaemophilic globulin). Only males are clinically affected, but females may act as carriers for the trait. The children of a normal male and a carrier female are on average 50 per cent normal, 25 per cent haemophilic males and 25 per cent carrier females; the children of a haemophilic male and a normal female are 50 per cent normal males and 50 per cent carrier females (Fig. 12).*

Haemophiliac patients usually give a family history of a bleeding tendency; but the condition sometimes arises, de novo, by mutation. The extent of the deficiency, and therefore the clinical severity of the condition, varies widely, but tends to breed true in any given family. A reduction of the plasma factor VIII concentration to 25 to 50 per cent of normal gives rise to severe bleeding following major trauma; a reduction to 10 per cent produces serious bleeding on minor trauma; while a complete deficiency of factor VIII is accompanied by spontaneous haemorrhage from the mucous membranes, and into the

---

*The union of a haemophilic male and a carrier female should theoretically give rise to children, of whom one in four is a haemophilic *female*. It was previously thought that this gene combination was lethal; a few cases of true female haemophilia have now, however, been recognized.

gastrointestinal and urinary tracts. Spontaneous haemorrhage characteristically occurs into the joints and muscles where it causes crippling deformities. Intravenously injectable factor VIII is now available for domiciliary use by the patient, and is revolutionising the lives of many haemophiliacs.

The bleeding time in haemophilia is normal. But, except in the mildest cases, there is prolongation of the clotting time *in vitro*. The thromboplastin generation test is almost always abnormal, a fact of diagnostic importance.

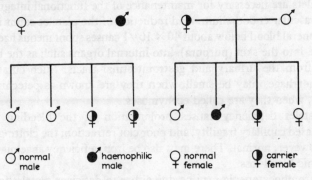

Fig. 12. Inheritance of haemophilia.

Factor VIII deficiency occurs also in von Willebrand's disease, which is an inherited condition affecting females as well as males.

Christmas disease
Christmas disease is a condition which is clinically very similar to haemophilia; in Britain, however, it is much less common. The deficiency is of factor IX (Christmas factor—named after the first family in England found to have this disease).

Afibrinogenaemia and the acute defibrination syndrome
In addition to a congenital or acquired defect in fibrinogen formation, a deficiency of this factor may arise from widespread intravascular clotting, as may follow retroplacental haemorrhage, or cardiopulmonary bypass (acute defibrination syndrome). Such intravascular coagulation seems to be initiated by the release of factor III into the general circulation, causing extensive fibrin deposition onto the vascular endothelium (where it is removed by the activity of fibrinolytic enzymes). There is thus a severe reduction of the circulating fibrinogen concentration, and consequently a tendency to prolonged haemorrhage from surgical incisions and after childbirth. Factors II, V and

VIII may also be reduced, although the administration of fibrinogen is usually sufficient to abolish the patient's coagulation defect.

A haemorrhagic tendency can arise also from the formation of excessive amounts of plasmin activator. Such a condition may occur following trauma, and in a variety of other conditions, including metastatic prostatic carcinoma, incompatible blood transfusion, and hepatic cirrhosis.

Platelet deficiency (thrombocytopenia)

Platelets are necessary for maintenance of the functional integrity of the vascular endothelium. And reduction of the platelet count in the peripheral blood below about $40 \times 10^9/1$ causes spontaneous haemorrhage into the skin (purpura), into internal organs such as the brain, and from the urinary and gastrointestinal tracts. Such cutaneous haemorrhages may be small, when they are known as petechiae, or large, when they are called ecchymoses.

Platelet deficiency causes prolongation of the bleeding time, increased capillary fragility, and poor clot retraction; the clotting time is, however, normal. There may also be iron deficiency anaemia from chronic blood loss.

Thrombocytopenia may be due either to deficient platelet formation, or to excessive platelet destruction, as accompanies the hypersplenism of hepatic cirrhosis (q.v.), Gaucher's disease and Felty's syndrome. Deficient formation may be 'idiopathic', or secondary to drug toxicity or neoplastic invasion of the bone-marrow. Thus, it may occur in leukaemia, lymphosarcoma or lymphadenoma, or when marrow function is depressed by the action of ionizing radiations. Certain drugs, such as chloramphenicol, tend to cause pancytopenia, with anaemia, agranulocytosis and thrombocytopenia; other drugs, such as sedormid, quinine and quinidine, cause a specific platelet deficiency, probably as a result of an antigen-antibody reaction. In this type of thrombocytopenia the bone marrow usually contains normal numbers of megakaryocytes.

Purpura occurs also in the absence of platelet deficiency (nonthrombocytopenic purpura), when the capillary wall is damaged by anaphylaxis (Henoch-Schönlein purpura), severe infection, or by the action of drugs or bacterial toxaemia. It may occur in scurvy, in old age when there is atrophy of the collagenous tissue supporting the capillaries (senile purpura), and in otherwise normal women (purpura simplex).

FURTHER READING

Anon 1976 von Willebrand's disease. British Medical Journal ii: 715

Aronstam A, Arblaster P G 1978 The haemolytic disorders including haemophilia. Practitioner 221: 176

Biggs R, MacFarlane R G 1962 Christmas disease. Post-Graduate Medical Journal 38: 3

British Medical Bulletin 1977 Haemostasis 33: 183

Campbell E J M, Dickinson C J, Slater J D H 1974 Clinical physiology, 4th edn. Blackwell, Oxford, ch 8

Dormandy K M 1968 Coagulation disorders. In: Baron D N, Compston N, Dawson A M (ed) Recent advances in medicine, 15th edn. Churchill, London

Eastham R D 1967 Practitioner 199: 29

Flute P J 1976 Thrombolytic therapy. British Journal of Hospital Medicine 16: 135

Hirsh J 1973 Bleeding disorders and fibrinolysis. In: Harvard CWH Frontiers of medicine, 3rd edn. Heinemann, London

Ingram G I C 1967 Current views on haemostasis. Practitioner 199: 5

MacFarlane R G 1964 An enzyme cascade in the blood clotting mechanism and its function as a biochemical amplifier. Nature, London 202: 498

Nilsson I M 1974 Haemorrhagic and thrombotic diseases, English edn. Wiley, Chichester

Thompson R B 1979 A short textbook of haematology, 5th edn. Pitman, London

7

Renal failure

A complex organism such as man can remain alive only if the composition of the fluid surrounding his tissue cells (the milieu intérieur of Claude Bernard*) is maintained constant. Such constancy of internal environment is achieved by the excretion of various metabolically-produced waste products and non-metabolized substances, ingested in excess of the body's needs. The body's chief excretory organ is the kidneys, which thus play a major role in tissue homeostasis; and depression of renal function gives rise to widespread biochemical abnormalities—the condition of renal failure. (The body's other major excretory organ is the lungs; the equivalent of some 12 500 mmol of hydrogen ions is eliminated each day in the expired air.)

When the kidneys fail adequately to perform their normal excretory function, various substances accumulate in the blood, and give rise to the clinical picture of renal failure. This condition may be acute or chronic. In acute renal failure the daily urine volume is reduced until it is no longer sufficient to eliminate the body's normal renal excretory load. In chronic failure the daily urine volume is usually relatively normal, but the concentrating ability of the kidneys is so impaired that this volume is insufficient to eliminate the body's waste products; metabolites and other substances therefore accumulate in the blood, causing clinical manifestations of chronic renal failure.

Although it is common practice to assess the severity of an individual patient's condition from the extent to which his blood urea concentration is raised, the symptoms of renal failure ('uraemia') are not due to urea retention *per se*, and there is a poor correlation between the patient's clinical condition and his blood urea concentration. There is evidence that the likely toxins lie mainly in the 'middle molecule range' i.e. mol. wt. 500–5000; but, in general, it may be said that many of the recognized biochemical abnormalities of renal failure produce no clinical manifestations; while, conversely, many of the

*Qu'est-ce que ce milieu intérieur? C'est le sang, non pas à la vérité le sang tout entier, mais la partie fluide du sang, le plasma sanguin, ensemble de tous liquides interstitiels, source et confluent de tous les échanges élémentaires' (Claude Bernard).

signs and symptoms of this condition have no well-defined biochemical basis.

PHYSIOLOGY

Urine is formed primarily by ultrafiltration of plasma in the renal glomeruli. The energy required for this process is provided by the hydrostatic pressure of the blood in the renal glomerular capillaries. As the filtrate passes down the nephron, it is modified by the addition and/or removal of various substances. Filtered water and electrolytes are partially reabsorbed from the proximal and distal tubules, and from the collecting ducts; glucose and potassium ions are removed almost completely from the proximal tubules; and other substances such as ammonia, hydrogen ions and potassium ions are secreted into the distal tubules.

Glomerular filtration
The two kidneys together receive about one-quarter of the resting cardiac output. Renal blood flow is therefore very high (about 1¼ l/min), a fact which is related not so much to the kidney's metabolic rate (renal oxygen extraction is the lowest in the body—only about 10 ml/l), as to their need to clear the blood of waste products.

The majority of the resistance to renal blood flow is provided by the efferent glomerular arterioles, very little by the afferent arterioles, therefore the hydrostatic pressure in the glomerular capillaries is relatively high (about 60 mmHg), and is sufficient to filter off a considerable proportion (about 20 per cent) of the glomerular plasma flow. Such filtration is opposed by the colloid osmotic pressure (oncotic pressure) of the plasma proteins, therefore, in conditions such as the nephrotic syndrome in which this pressure is reduced, the glomerular filtration rate may be considerably above normal. In a fit, healthy adult the glomerular filtration rate is approximately 120 ml/min, although it declines somewhat with age (as do many other physiological parameters). The ratio of glomerular filtration rate to renal plasma flow is known as the filtration fraction.

The glomerular filter is formed mainly by the basement membrane which separates the glomerular capillary endothelium from the tubular endothelium of Bowman's capsule. This membrane readily permits the passage of molecules smaller than about 60000, but is almost completely impermeable to larger molecules, such as those of the plasma proteins. The glomerular filtrate is thus an ultrafiltrate of the plasma, and (apart from slight differences due to the Donnan effect), contains small molecules, such as glucose, urea, etc., in the same concentration as does the plasma, but larger molecules, such as protein, hardly at all. (The concentration of protein in the glomerular filtrate is normally about 200 mg/l, cf. the normal plasma protein concentration of 70g/l.)

Some 170 litres of glomerular filtrate are formed each day, whereas in the same period the normal rate of urine excretion is only one or two litres; and, even under conditions of extreme diuresis, the daily urinary output does not exceed 10 litres.

Proximal tubular function

Some four-fifths of the glomerular filtrate is reabsorbed by the cells of the proximal tubules. In addition, certain substances, such as glucose, which are of particular value to the economy of the body, are actively reabsorbed from this region of the nephron, more or less completely. (An active process is one which requires the expenditure of metabolically-produced energy, cf. a passive process such as diffusion or osmosis.)

The main driving force for the reabsorption of water and electrolytes from the proximal tubules is the active transport of sodium ions out of the tubular lumen. Sodium ions are, of course, positively charged, therefore their movement out of the tubule causes a potential difference between the tubular lumen and the surrounding extracellular fluid; negatively-charged chloride ions move out of the tubule along this electrical potential gradient. And, since the endothelial lining of the proximal tubules is permeable to water, water is osmotically reabsorbed with the sodium and chloride ions, maintaining the tubular fluid roughly isotonic with the plasma.

Impairment of sodium reabsorption by the tubular endothelium, as by the action of mercurial or other diuretics, causes increased fluid and electrolyte loss from the body (diuresis). Diuresis occurs also when osmotically active material in the tubular lumen hinders water reabsorption (osmotic diuresis); this occurs, for example, with glucose in diabetes mellitus (q.v.), and when non-metabolizable sugars, such as mannitol, are administered intravenously.

Glucose is actively reabsorbed from the proximal tubule, and is normally absent from the distal tubular fluid, and from the urine itself. There is, however, a limit to the rate at which glucose can be transported across the tubular endothelium, and, when this rate is exceeded, glucose appears in the urine (glycosuria—see section on diabetes mellitus). The maximum rate of glucose reabsorption is known as the tubular maximum for glucose, Tm_G, and is normally in the region of 350 mg/min.

If all nephrons were identical, with a total glomerular filtration rate of 120 ml/min, the Tm_G would be exceeded at a plasma glucose concentration of about $350 \times 100/120 \simeq 300$ mg/100 ml (16.7 mmol/1). However, it is well recognized clinically that, with normal renal function, glycosuria occurs when the plasma glucose concentration exceeds a much lower value, e.g. 180 mg/100 ml (10.0 mmol/1). The reason for this anomaly is that the ratio of glomerular filtration to tubular reabsorptive ability varies from nephron to nephron; and the Tm_G of a nephron with relatively poor absorptive ability is exceeded at a relatively low glucose concentration.

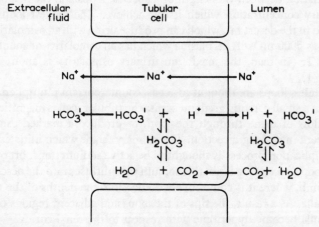

Fig. 13. Reabsorption of bicarbonate ions from proximal renal tubule.

Potassium ions also are actively reabsorbed from the proximal tubule, so that they are absent from the fluid entering the distal part of the nephron. (The potassium which appears in the urine is resecreted into the distal tubule, in exchange for sodium—see later.)

Bicarbonate ions are removed from the proximal tubular fluid, roughly in proportion to water reabsorption. Bicarbonate reabsorption depends on the activity of the enzyme, carbonic anhydrase, which is present in the brush borders of the proximal tubular cells. Bicarbonate ions, being charged, pass through the tubular endothelium with difficulty; in the tubular lumen, however, they are able to combine with hydrogen ions to form carbonic acid,

$$HCO'_3 + H^+ \rightleftharpoons H_2CO_3$$

and in the presence of carbonic anhydrase, H_2CO_3 dissociates into water and carbon dioxide (Fig. 13). Carbon dioxide, being a gas, is readily diffusible and can thus pass through the tubular endothelium into the peritubular capillaries, hence the expression 'bicarbonate ions are absorbed in the form of carbon dioxide'.

There is in fact a fall of pH (to about 7.0) down the length of the proximal tubule, indicating that hydrogen ion secretion is in excess of bicarbonate absorption.

Loops of Henle

It is now appreciated that the loops of Henle—the function of which was long a mystery—are concerned chiefly with urinary concentration. Loops of Henle are possessed only by those phyla which produce a urine hypertonic in relation to the plasma; also, there is a strong correlation between the length of a species' loops and the maximum urinary concentration which it can achieve. The longest loops are found in the desert rat, which can produce urine with an osmolarity as high as 5000 mOs/1, cf. plasma which has an osmolarity of about 300 mOs/1. (In man, the maximum urinary osmolarity is about 1300 mOs/1).

Henle's loops are thought to act as 'countercurrent multipliers', by which a small osmotic gradient across the tubular wall is magnified by the flow of urine through the loop, to produce a marked osmotic gradient in its long direction. The primary factor which initiates this multiplication process is thought to be active sodium transport out of the loop's ascending limb; this sodium then diffuses into the descending limb, where it is convectively carried into the depths of the renal medulla. As a result, the tips of the loops and adjacent regions of the medulla become hypertonic with respect to the renal cortex.

(The vasa recta are, of course, also arranged in a countercurrent manner. They probably act as osmotic countercurrent exchangers, the function of which is to minimize the effect of the medullary blood flow on the hyperosmolarity of this region of the kidney. Lever (see recommended further reading) has, however, recently suggested that the vasa recta may act primarily as countercurrent *multipliers*, i.e. that they are responsible for *generating* medullary hyperosmolarity, as well as for its maintenance.)

The distal tubules

In the distal convoluted tubules the composition of the urine is adjusted finally in accordance with the needs of the body. Proximal tubular function appears to be largely 'obligatory', i.e. invariant; the distal parts of the nephron are, however, under hormonal control, and their function varies widely, according to circumstances.

As a result of the transfer of sodium ions out of the ascending limb of Henle's loop (see above), the fluid at the start of the distal tubules is hypotonic with respect to the plasma. In the presence of antidiuretic hormone (ADH—see section on water balance), however, the distal tubular endothelium becomes permeable to water, so that the tubular contents become isotonic with the plasma. In the absence of ADH the endothelium remains relatively impermeable to water; in consequence, the urine remains hypotonic, and, indeed, becomes progressively more so as sodium reabsorption continues along the tubule.

Distal sodium reabsorption is accompanied by transfer of chloride ions, and by sodium/potassium exchange across the tubular endothelium. This exchange occurs under the influence of aldosterone, secreted by the adrenal cortex (see Chapter 10). In the absence of such aldosterone secretion some 2 per cent of the filtered sodium is excreted in the urine; under maximum aldosterone activity, however, tubular sodium is almost completely absorbed. Excessive aldosterone activity, such as occurs in Cushing's syndrome, results in enhanced sodium/potassium exchange, with consequent sodium retention and loss of excessive amounts of potassium in the urine. Conversely, in adrenal cortical hypofunction (Addison's disease—q.v.) there is excessive urinary sodium loss, with depletion of the extracellular fluid volume (see sections on sodium balance and potassium retention).

When the body is producing an acid urine, as is normally the case, there is also active hydrogen ion transport into the lumen of the distal tubule (see below). This process appears to involve the same mechanism as does the transport of potassium ions; potassium and hydrogen ions are thus in competition, and the reduced hydrogen ion transfer which occurs in alkalosis may so enhance potassium excretion as to cause potassium deficiency (q.v.).

(If, as is commonly the case, the alkalosis results from prolonged vomiting, there is an accompanying reduction of extracellular fluid volume. This hypovolaemia stimulates aldosterone secretion, and thus enhances sodium/potassium and sodium/hydrogen ion exchange across the tubular walls, with aggravation of the renal potassium loss, and the paradoxical production of an acid urine—see section on pyloric stenosis.)

Role in acid-base regulation*

It is in the distal part of the nephron also that the composition of the urine is adjusted in accordance with the body's acid-base requirements. On a normal diet, the body has to excrete in the urine about 100 mmol of hydrogen ions per day, derived mainly from protein metabolism. There is, however, a limit to the hydrogen ion concentration which can be achieved in the distal tubular fluid—a pH of about 4.5, which corresponds to a free hydrogen ion concentration of about 0.03 mmol/l—and, without the presence of urinary buffers, the

*The basic terminology of acid-base physiology is explained in Chapter 12

excretion of this hydrogen ion load would require a daily urine output of some 3000 litres! Fortunately, although the maximum acidity of the urine is fixed, the number of hydrogen ions excreted can be increased many times by buffering, chiefly with phosphate ions and ammonia (Fig. 14).

When the kidneys are producing an acid urine, the bicarbonate ions which reach the distal tubules are quickly combined with hydrogen ions; but there remains a quantity of phosphate which is able to buffer hydrogen ions according to the equation:

$$H^+ + HPO''_4 \rightleftharpoons H_2PO'_4.$$

This reaction considerably increases the number of hydrogen ions which can be excreted at a given urinary pH.

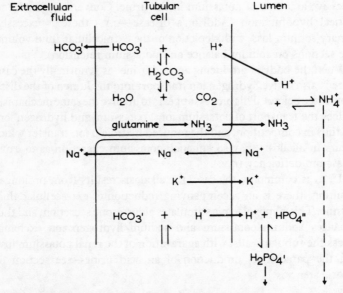

Fig. 14. Buffering of hydrogen ions in distal renal tubule.

Hydrogen ions are buffered also by combination with ammonia. This is formed by the enzymatic conversion of glutamine and other amines in the tubular cells, from where it diffuses into the tubular lumen to combine with hydrogen ions according to the equation:

$$H^+ + NH_3 \rightleftharpoons NH^+_4.$$

Ammonium ions, being electrically charged and therefore unable to diffuse back across the tubular membrane, are excreted in the urine.

Concentration and dilution of the urine

The way in which the permeability of the distal tubular endothelium depends on the presence or absence of ADH has already been considered. In the absence of ADH, the urine remains hypotonic during its passage along the distal tubules and collecting ducts, and is excreted in a dilute, hypotonic form. With normal renal function, the specific gravity of the urine may fall very low, with a total osmolarity of about 30 mOs/1. In the presence of ADH the endothelium of the distal tubule and collecting ducts becomes permeable to water, which is extracted osmotically into the hypertonic interstitial tissue of the renal medulla, leaving the urine with a concentration of up to four times that of the plasma (specific gravity up to 1.030, osmolarity about 1,300 mOs/1). The water which is thus osmotically attracted into the medulla is carried away by the vasa recta.

Endocrine function of the kidneys

In addition to their homeostatic and excretory functions, the kidneys act as endocrine organs: they produce the hormone erythropoietin (see section on blood formation), and the enzyme renin, which is concerned with the formation of angiotensin from angiotensinogen (see section on hypertension); and they are concerned with the conversion of 25-hydroxycalciferol into the active metabolite 1,25-dihydroxycalciferol (see section on calcium balance).

ACUTE RENAL FAILURE

Acute renal failure is accompanied usually by a severe reduction of urine volume (anuria or oliguria), and therefore by inability of the kidneys to eliminate the body's metabolic end-products. This function normally requires a urine volume of around 700 ml/day; but considerably more when renal concentrating ability is impaired (see Fig. 21 and section on water balance). The initial stages of recovery from renal failure may be accompanied by considerable diuresis; renal concentrating power is then so poor that, despite an increased urine output, the kidneys are unable to excrete the solute load presented to them; renal failure then occurs even in the absence of oliguria.

The oliguria of renal failure from acute tubular necrosis (see below) is accompanied by a reduction of renal blood flow to about one-third of normal. Glomerular filtration rate, as measured by standard techniques, is reduced to as low as 1 per cent of normal. (This figure is, however, probably inaccurate, because the damaged tubules permit substances, filtered by the glomeruli, to leak back into the peritubular capillaries; therefore inulin and creatinine clearance rates no longer give valid estimates of the glomerular filtration rate.)

In some conditions, e.g. severe glomerulonephritis, urine volume is reduced virtually to zero. In tubular necrosis it is in the region of 50 to 100 ml/day, and the urine is dark from the presence of necrosed tubular cells. In acute renal failure from glomerulonephritis or 'pre-renal uraemia' (see below and Chapter 2) the urine is concentrated as a result of ADH activity; the damaged tubules of acute tubular necrosis are, however, unable to respond to this hormone and, despite its 'concentrated' appearance, the urine has a specific gravity of around 1.010, i.e. the same as the plasma.

ETIOLOGY

Acute renal failure may result from mechanical factors, as when the urinary tract is blocked by calculi or bilateral ureteric obstruction from some other cause. It occurs also in patients with severe acute glomeru-lonephritis, or other form of intrinsic renal disease. Most commonly, however, the condition arises directly or indirectly as a result of renal circulatory impairment.

A severe reduction of extracellular fluid volume, e.g. as a result of prolonged vomiting, may cause a fall in renal blood flow and a consequent impairment of renal function. This is the condition of pre-renal uraemia.

In hypovolaemic shock (q.v.) there is a reduction of renal blood flow as the body attempts to divert its reduced cardiac output towards essential organs, such as the brain and heart. There is in consequence a severe reduction of glomerular filtration, with marked oliguria; and such urine as is produced is concentrated by the action of ADH, secreted in response to the hypovolaemia (see section on water balance). Provided the physiological disturbance responsible for the patient's acute reduction of renal perfusion is promptly treated, renal function is rapidly restored; but if the condition is permitted to persist untreated for more than a few hours the kidneys may be damaged so severely that the failure becomes potentially irreversible—the condi-tion of acute tubular necrosis.

Acute tubular necrosis may be caused also by incompatible blood transfusion, severe infection, and by the action of poisons such as mercury, arsenic and carbon tetrachloride. Tubular necrosis from the action of toxins tends to affect preferentially the proximal tubules; whereas renal ischaemia tends to cause patchy areas of necrosis involving the whole nephron.

BIOCHEMICAL ABNORMALITIES

The oliguria of acute renal failure is accompanied by retention of a variety of metabolites and waste products, and by disturbances of fluid and electrolyte balance. Potassium retention is particularly likely to cause symptoms, and may result in fatal ventricular fibrillation.

Water

The excretion of water is not a great problem in acute renal failure. Even in the presence of complete anuria there is still a net loss from the body of about 500 ml/day—500 ml lost from the lungs, 500 ml lost as insensible perspiration, and 500 ml gained as a result of fat and carbohydrate metabolism. Complete water restriction is thus unnecessary. However, if the patient's water intake is not reduced in line with his reduced urinary output he may develop hyponatraemia and signs of 'water intoxication' (see section on water balance), with headache, confusion and even convulsions. This situation may be aggravated by misguided attempts to 'flush out the patient's kidneys' by the oral or intravenous administration of large amounts of hypotonic fluid. (Of course, this is not to say that fluids should always be withheld from patients with acute renal failure; restoration of blood volume in a shocked patient suffering from pre-renal uraemia rapidly restores renal function, and is an important prophylactic measure against the development of acute tubular necrosis.)

Electrolytes and other solutes

Acute renal failure is accompanied by retention of a variety of substances—urea, creatinine, potassium, phosphate, sulphate and other anions, and hydrogen ions. For any given reduction of glomerular filtration rate the blood urea concentration depends on the rate of protein catabolism (Fig. 15), which in turn depends on the amount of protein contained in the patient's diet and on the rate of tissue breakdown. Renal failure is commonly accompanied by increased tissue metabolism ('hypercatabolism'), as a result of trauma, infection or involution of the gravid uterus; under these circumstances the blood urea concentration rises markedly, and rapidly. The catabolism of 100 g of protein yields approximately 30 g of urea, which, if accumulated in a total body water of, say, 50 l, would cause the blood urea concentration to rise by some 60 mg/100ml (10 mmol/1).

Increased metabolism increases also the renal excretory loads of potassium, phosphate and hydrogen ions. The resulting increase of plasma potassium concentration (hyperkalaemia) is likely to have serious consequences; and may be aggravated by concomitant

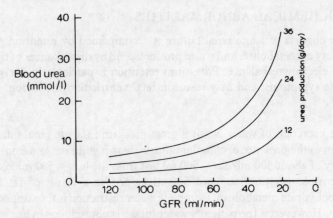

Fig. 15. Dependence of blood urea concentration on glomerular filtration rate (GFR) for different rates of urea production (g/24 h). Urea clearance assumed to be 60 per cent of GFR. Note hyperbolic relationship between blood urea concentration and GFR.

hypoxia, which impairs the efficiency of the cellular 'sodium pump' (thus permitting potassium ions to diffuse out into the plasma), and by acidosis, which causes hydrogen ions to move intracellularly so displacing potassium ions into the plasma.

Increase of plasma phosphate concentration may reciprocally lower its calcium concentration, and may even result in tetany.

Hydrogen ion retention causes a metabolic (non-respiratory) acidosis, and deep, sighing respirations, known clinically as Kussmaul breathing or 'air hunger'. Physiologically, the explanation for the patient's alveolar hyperventilation is that the increase of plasma hydrogen ion concentration stimulates pulmonary ventilation, and thus, by reducing the P_{CO_2} of the arterial blood restores the plasma pH towards normal. The patient's primary metabolic acidosis is compensated by a respiratory alkalosis (Figs. 16 and 17, and Chapter 12).

Increase of plasma potassium concentration impairs the contractile ability of both skeletal and cardiac muscle. It also causes characteristic e.c.g. changes (see section on potassium balance). Severe elevation of the plasma potassium concentration may result in ventricular fibrillation, and is an indication for renal dialysis (see page 96).

CLINICAL MANIFESTATIONS OF ACUTE RENAL FAILURE

Acute renal failure is accompanied in its early stages by few clinical manifestations, except for a rapidly developing and progressive anaemia. However, if the condition remains untreated for more than a

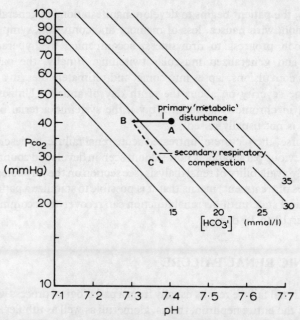

Fig. 16. Compensated and uncompensated metabolic (non-respiratory) acidosis, plotted on Siggaard-Andersen nomogram, (see Chapter 12). Point A—normal acid-base state ($P\mathrm{CO}_2 = 40$ mmHg (5.3 k Pa) pH = 7.40); point B—uncompensated metabolic acidosis; point C—compensated metabolic acidosis.

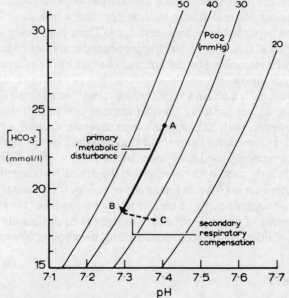

Fig. 17. As Figure 16, but plotted on Davenport diagram.

few days, the patient begins to develop manifestations of generalized intoxication, with nausea, loss of memory and confusion, symptoms which soon progress to drowsiness, accompanied by hyperactive reflexes and generalized muscular twitching. Finally, the patient develops convulsions, lapses into coma, and ultimately dies (in a case of average severity on about the tenth day of anuria). Unlike the situation in chronic renal failure (q.v.), the systemic arterial blood pressure is not usually raised.

Of course, the picture of untreated acute renal failure, as described in the previous paragraph, is now seldom seen in developed countries. The ready availability of renal dialysis (see section on the physiological principles of treatment) means that it is possible to stabilize a patient's biochemical state until his renal function can recover, as it commonly does after 10 to 14 days.

CHRONIC RENAL FAILURE

Chronic renal failure results usually from a pathological process which damages the entire nephron, that is, glomeruli as well as tubules. As a result, there is a progressive reduction in the number of functioning nephrons, with impairment of renal function, until ultimately the kidneys become unable to maintain the composition of the internal environment within limits which are compatible with life. Clinical manifestations of renal failure become apparent when some 75 per cent of the nephrons have been destroyed. There is however a great reserve of renal function; and with appropriate dietary measures life of a sort may be maintained by the function of as little as 2 per cent of the nephron population.

Chronic renal failure has a varied etiology; but the end result is fairly constant, and gives rise to the clinical picture of 'uraemia'. It should be noted, however, that, although the term uraemia is almost synonymous with chronic renal failure, and although the blood urea concentration is commonly used as an index of the severity of an individual patient's failure, there is no evidence that the clinical manifestations of this condition are due to urea retention *per se*. Indeed, the intravenous injection of large amounts of urea in no way reproduces the clinical manifestations of uraemia, which are thought to be due mainly to the retention of other (in the main unidentified) metabolites (see earlier).

ETIOLOGY

Chronic renal failure may result from a variety of pathological processes. It may accompany primary renal disease, such as chronic glomerulonephritis, chronic pyelonephritis, and polycystic disease. It occurs also when the kidneys are damaged by drugs such as phenacetin,* by generalized disease processes, such as disseminated lupus erythematosus, polyarteritis nodosa, amyloid disease, and endocrine abnormalities, such as diabetes mellitus and hypercalcaemia, and it may accompany systemic hypertension (q.v.) both benign and malignant, and chronic obstruction of the urinary tract as a result of, for example, urethral stricture, prostatic hypertrophy, and bilateral ureteric obstruction.

BIOCHEMICAL ABNORMALITIES

Patients with chronic renal failure have impaired renal concentrating ability, with polyuria and nocturnal frequency of micturition. They suffer also from retention of a variety of metabolites, including urea, uric acid (may precipitate an acute attack of gout), creatinine, phenolic compounds and various amines.

Water

One of the early and important signs of deteriorating renal function is impairment of renal concentrating ability, necessitating an increased urine output to excrete a given solute load (see Chapter 12 and Fig. 21). This defect of renal function is manifested initially by loss of the normal diurnal variation in urine concentration, and by consequent nocturnal frequency of micturition (nocturia). In severe cases there is increased urine formation throughout the 24 hours (polyuria), but not as great as that found in diabetes mellitus and diabetes insipidus. Ultimately, the kidneys lose also their ability to produce a dilute urine, with the result that the urine comes to have a fixed osmolarity, equal to that of the plasma (isosthenuria).

The damaged kidneys' inability to concentrate the urine seems to be related mainly to reduction in the total number of functioning nephrons. Provided the patient is taking a normal diet, the amount of osmotically-active solutes to be excreted is roughly the same as in a normal person; the number of nephrons is, however, considerably reduced, therefore the solute load per nephron is above normal. The passage of this increased solute load down the nephron is thought to induce an osmotic diuresis, rather analogous to that found in diabetes mellitus (q.v.).

In addition, patients with chronic renal failure may have renal

*Until recently phenacetin was a common ingredient of a variety of proprietary analgesic tablets.

medullary fibrosis, or an abnormality of the ratio of cortical to medullary blood flow. The operation of the medullary counter-current multiplier (see earlier) is thus impaired, causing a reduction of hypertonicity in this region of the kidney and a consequent impairment of renal concentrating ability.

Even when the failing kidneys are still able to produce a dilute urine, their ability to excrete a large water load is impaired. The maximum rate of urine flow in a patient with chronic renal failure seldom exceeds 3 or 4 l/day (cf. the normal figure of about 8 litres).

Hydrogen ions

On a normal diet, the kidneys must excrete some 100 to 150 mmol of hydrogen ions per day, if the internal environment is not to become excessively acid. The urine is therefore normally on the acid side of neutrality, and contains considerable quantities of hydrogen ions, most of which are excreted in combination with the buffers, ammonia and phosphate.

(The normal minimum urinary pH is about 4.5. This corresponds to a free hydrogen ion concentration of only about 0.03 mmol/1. At this pH, the titratable acidity of the urine—the amount of alkali required to titrate it to a neutral pH, i.e. to neutralize both free hydrogen ions and those combined with phosphate and other buffers—is of the order of 70 mmol/1. In addition, a considerable number of hydrogen ions are excreted combined with ammonia).

In chronic renal failure the ability of the kidneys to excrete hydrogen ions is considerably reduced; they therefore accumulate in the plasma, causing a metabolic acidosis* (see section on acute renal failure). Such inability to excrete hydrogen ions is due in part to reduction of the rate at which the distal renal tubules can produce ammonia from glutamine and other amines, and in part to unknown factors. There is no impairment of the kidneys' ability to lower the urinary pH, only of their capacity to excrete hydrogen ions in combination with ammonia and other buffers.

The reduction of plasma bicarbonate concentration which occurs in renal failure is accompanied by retention of sulphate and other anions. These maintain the electrical neutrality of the plasma, and thus obviate the need for chloride retention, such as occurs in some other forms of metabolic acidosis—'hyperchloraemic acidosis'.

Electrolyte imbalance

Severe abnormalities of sodium and potassium balance are uncommon

---

*The severity of a patient's metabolic acidosis is determined by measuring the so-called 'standard bicarbonate concentration' of his plasma—see section on acid-base balance.

in chronic renal failure until the final stages of the disease. There is, however, usually impairment of the body's ability to deal with a sudden alteration of sodium and/or potassium intake. Terminal renal failure may be accompanied by marked potassium retention.

Occasionally, patients with impaired renal function have, despite increased aldosterone secretion, an abnormal, and inappropriate, renal sodium loss. This is the condition of 'salt-losing nephritis.'

Calcium and phosphorus
In chronic renal failure, there is commonly defective absorption of calcium from the gut, and the rate of urinary calcium excretion may be considerably below normal, perhaps as low as 10 mg/day (cf. the average normal figure of 100 mg/day). There is also resistance to the action of vitamin D, although the bony lesions which accompany such hypocalcaemia may be ameliorated or cured by the administration of dietary calcium supplements and large doses of this vitamin (see section on osteomalacia). In some patients the impairment of calcium absorption is sufficiently severe to cause hypocalcaemia, and even overt tetany.

There is also commonly a raised plasma phosphate concentration due to the reduced glomerular filtration rate, although in the early stages of renal failure increased PTH secretion may, by reducing tubular phosphate reabsorption, be able to maintain a normal plasma phosphate level. In some patients the increased parathyroid secretion causes the development of osteitis fibrosa (see section on hyperparathyroidism). Such patients have a normal, or slightly raised, plasma calcium concentration. (The finding of a markedly raised plasma calcium level in a patient with renal failure suggests that his condition is the *result*, rather than the cause, of his high plasma calcium concentration, i.e. that his renal failure is secondary to hypercalcaemia from e.g. endocrine-secreting tumours, osteolytic metastatic deposits, or primary hyperparathyroidism (q.v.).

Magnesium
In chronic renal failure there is usually reduced magnesium absorption. Magnesium excretion is, however, reduced also, so that the body's magnesium balance is approximately normal, although its ability to deal with an increased magnesium load is impaired. The administration of a magnesium sulphate purge to a patient with chronic renal failure may have fatal consequences.

Anaemia
Patients with chronic renal failure are anaemic, roughly in proportion

to the height of their blood urea concentration. Anaemia also develops rapidly in acute renal failure. The reduction of haemoglobin concentration in both conditions is due to several factors, the chief of which is probably bone marrow depression from generalized 'toxaemia', and from the damaged kidneys' inability to produce erythropoietin (see section on anaemia). In addition, red cell survival time may be shortened, so that the anaemia has a haemolytic element; while, terminally, the patient may develop a bleeding tendency with the result that the anaemia is aggravated by blood loss.

CLINICAL MANIFESTATIONS OF CHRONIC RENAL FAILURE

Gastrointestinal

Uraemic patients usually experience gastrointestinal symptoms, such an anorexia, nausea and vomiting, and in consequence tend to lose weight and become emaciated; persistent hiccough is also common.

Terminally, there is a tendency to gastrointestinal haemorrhage, with haematemesis and/or melaena. The resulting hypovolaemia may have serious consequences, because it reduces renal blood flow (see section on shock) and glomerular filtration rate, and thus exacerbates the renal failure. Also, the blood in the gastrointestinal tract is equivalent to a large protein meal, and therefore imposes a severe nitrogenous load on the damaged kidneys.

Neurological

The neurological manifestations of chronic renal failure tend to be relatively non-specific, with headache, lassitude and generalized muscular weakness. Terminally, the patient may become confused, and finally comatose. Fits occur occasionally; and muscular twitching is common, apparently the result of spontaneous and irregular discharge of anterior horn cells in the spinal cord.

There may also be peripheral neuropathy, with paraesthesiae and paresis of the extremities, particularly of the legs.

Cardiovascular

Renal failure and hypertension (q.v.) are intimately associated, because, not only may renal disease cause hypertension, but hypertension from a non-renal cause tends, sooner or later, to impair renal function (nephrosclerosis). The initial changes in this condition affect the renal vasculature; later they produce ischaemic changes in the nephrons, similar to those seen in chronic renal failure from other causes. In malignant hypertension (q.v.) there is rapid obliteration of the vascular lumen from endarteritis and fibrinoid necrosis of the vessel wall.

In addition, renal failure may be accompanied by other cardiovascular changes, such as aseptic pericarditis of unknown etiology, and changes in the lungs resembling pulmonary oedema ('uraemic lung'). This latter condition appears to be due partly to pulmonary congestion, consequent on hypertensive left heart failure (q.v.), and partly to increased pulmonary capillary permeability.

Cutaneous

Chronic renal failure may cause cutaneous pigmentation which, in conjunction with the patient's anaemia, may produce a pale, dirty beige discoloration of the skin. There may also be non-thrombocytopenic purpura from widespread capillary damage. Cutaneous infections (boils, carbuncles, etc.) are common, and superficial abrasions tend to heal slowly.

Skeletal

A reduction of renal function causes hyperphosphataemia with or without a reduction of plasma calcium concentration and resistance to the action of vitamin D (see p. 139). The resulting effect on bone mineralization and formation seems to depend on *inter alia* the patient's intake of calcium, phosphorus, and vitamin D. Renal osteodystrophy may have features of osteomalacia, osteoporosis, osteosclerosis, or osteitis fibrosa (see Chapter 11).

PHYSIOLOGICAL PRINCIPLES OF TREATMENT

In untreated acute renal failure, toxic substances accumulate in the blood, until ultimately the patient is poisoned by the products of his own metabolism. In the presence of a virtually complete cessation of renal function, such as occurs in acute tubular necrosis (q.v.), death ensues, in the untreated patient, in about ten days. But if the patient can be kept alive until renal function begins to improve, there is every prospect that his renal function will eventually recover sufficiently for him to be able to lead an entirely normal life.

In the past the methods available for treating patients (see below) with acute tubular necrosis were ineffective, and the mortality from this condition was in excess of 90 per cent. With the development of techniques for peritoneal dialysis and haemodialysis, however, the mortality from acute renal failure has been reduced to below 25 per cent or better in special centres.

The results of the treatment of chronic renal failure are less encouraging. Some patients, such as those with renal failure from chronic pyelonephritis, can be improved by appropriate antibiotic treatment; but, in the majority, the condition is progressive, and ultimately fatal. In recent years, considerable success has been achieved in treating this condition by intermittent extracorporeal haemodialysis or renal transplantation. The problems are, however, still considerable, particularly so in view of the large numbers of patients who stand to benefit from such treatment.

Acute renal failure

Before the introduction of techniques for artificial haemodialysis, the cornerstone of the management of acute renal failure was maintenance of fluid and electrolyte balance, coupled with minimization of tissue metabolism by a high-carbohydrate, low-protein diet. The rationale for giving the patient's energy intake mainly in the form of carbohydrate was, of course, that it minimized protein metabolism, which would otherwise produce toxic end-products, such as potassium ions, hydrogen ions and various nitrogenous metabolites (including urea). At one time it was thought desirable to maintain the patient's energy intake by the administration of large quantities of fat (calorific value 9 Cal/g (37 kJ/g) cf. 4 Cal/g (17 kJ/g) for carbohydrate), but such a regime tends to cause gastrointestinal upset, and is no longer recommended.

It is possible by such dietary means to tide a patient over a brief episode of acute renal failure, particularly if this is not associated with hypercatabolism from injury, infection, etc. But, if the failure is severe or prolonged, dietary treatment must be supplemented by some form of artificial dialysis.

As a general rule, a patient whose blood urea is rising relatively slowly—at less than, say 5 mmol/l (30 mg/100 ml) per day—is likely to recover spontaneously before his biochemical derangement becomes sufficiently severe to necessitate dialysis; a critically injured patient with a rapidly rising blood urea concentration, however, is likely to need dialysis after only a few days' anuria.

The blood urea level at which artificial dialysis is instituted must (as always) be assessed in the light of the patient's clinical state, but is somewhere around a blood urea concentration of 33 mmol/l (200 mg/100 ml) in an adult, and considerably lower in a child.

Severe electrolyte losses may occur during recovery from acute renal failure, because the damaged kidneys' response to hormonal control is still impaired. In these circumstances care must be taken to prevent fluid and/or electrolyte depletion.

Dialysis

Artificial dialysis, as used in the treatment of acute renal failure, may be in the form of peritoneal dialysis or as haemodialysis using an extracorporeal 'artificial kidney'. The physiochemical principle of both these techniques is that the patient's blood is separated from the dialysing fluid by a thin membrane, which is readily permeable to small molecules, such as glucose, urea etc., but impermeable to larger molecules, such as plasma proteins, and to the cellular elements of the blood.

Diffusion across such a membrane occurs down the appropriate concentration gradient; therefore, by adjustment of the composition of the dialysing fluid, it is possible to transfer substances both into and out of the patient's blood. For example, if the dialysing fluid contains a low (or zero) concentration of urea this molecule will diffuse out of the blood, thus reducing the patient's blood urea concentration; while, if the concentration of sodium is the same on both sides of the membrane, no net transfer of this ion occurs. By making the dialysing fluid a hypertonic glucose solution, it is possible osmotically to remove water from the patient, and thus to reduce the danger of water intoxication (q.v.) in an overhydrated patient. (Glucose diffuses in the opposite direction, but is rapidly metabolized in the body, where it has a valuable protein-sparing effect.)

The dialysing membrane for peritoneal dialysis is provided by the endothelial lining of the abdominal cavity. An aliquot of dialysing fluid is run in via a nylon catheter, left in contact with the peritoneum for a short time, and then run out again to be replaced with fresh fluid. This process can be repeated many times with little discomfort to the patient, even in the presence of active peritonitis.

With extracorporeal haemodialysis the dialysing membrane is an artificial one, composed of cellophane or other synthetic material. Blood is led to the kidney machine from a superficial artery, and then, after flowing over the dialysing membrane, is returned to a convenient vein; a continuous flow of blood can thus be dialysed and cleared of toxic metabolites.

Chronic renal failure

It is now possible, by intermittent haemodialysis or renal transplantation, to reverse the biochemical abnormalities of chronic renal failure, and to keep patients with this condition alive for at least several years, and probably much longer. Intermittent haemodialysis has been greatly simplified by the use of arteriovenous fistulae, either external or subcutaneous and by the development of artificial kidneys which have only a small priming volume, and which do not require a separate pump. Patients are now increasingly being dialysed in their own homes, with the minimum of medical supervision and with a considerable reduction in the danger of their attendants' contracting viral hepatitis—a hazard which has caused havoc in many hospital dialysis units.

A promising new technique is haemofiltration in which an ultrafiltrate of the plasma is forced through an artificial membrane by hydrostatic pressure, and the fluid replaced by an infusion of Ringer lactate solution. The efficiency of this process at removing 'middle-range' molecules far exceeds that of the standard dialysis technique (insulin clearance 60 ml/min cf. 9 ml/min with conventional dialysis).

The best treatment for chronic renal failure is theoretically replacement of the damaged organ with the kidney of a dead donor. However, although the technical problems of renal transplantation are reasonably straightforward, there are great difficulties in arranging a satisfactory supply of donated organs; and the problem of immunological rejection is a bar to the long-term success of this technique. It is possible to minimize graft rejection by immunosuppressive techniques, but these are costly in medical resources and unpleasant to the patient. Also, it is being increasingly realized that there is an increased incidence of malignant disease in such patients, presumably because malignant mutant cells are no longer held in check by the body's normal immune responses. It is hoped that the use of computers to carefully match prospective donors and recipients may improve matters in the future; but the full benefits of this technique will be realized only when there are changes in the law relating to the removal of organs from the recently-dead.

FURTHER READING

Anon 1975 Anaemia in chronic renal failure. Lancet i: 959
Anon 1977 New technique for the treatment of endstage renal failure. British Medical Journal ii: 211
Anon 1977 What causes toxicity in uraemia. British Medical Journal ii: 143
Anon 1978 Hyperparathyroidism in renal failure. British Medical Journal i: 390
Anon 1978 Uraemia, azotaemia, sharks and camels. Lancet i: 421
Berlyne G M 1968 A course in renal diseases, 2nd edn. Blackwell, Oxford
Cameron J S 1966 Renal disease. British Medical Journal ii: 811, 873
Campbell E J M, Dickinson C J, Slater J D H 1974 Clinical physiology, 4th edn. Blackwell, Oxford, ch 4
de Wardener H E 1973 The kidney: an outline of normal and abnormal structure and function, 4th edn. Churchill, London
Evans D B 1977 Management of chronic renal failure by dialysis and transplantation. British Medical Journal i: 1585
Evans D B 1978 Acute renal failure. British Journal of Hospital Medicine 19: 197
Gamble J L 1954 Chemical anatomy, physiology and pathology of extracellular fluid, 6th edn. Harvard University Press, Cambridge, Mass.

Hoffman W S 1970 The biochemistry of clinical medicine, 4th edn. Year Book Medical Publishers, Chicago, ch 7, 8

Hosking D J 1977 Diseases of the urinary system: renal osteodystrophy. British Medical Journal ii: 110

Kerr D N S 1973 Management of chronic renal failure. In: Baron D N, Compston N, Dawson A M (ed) Recent advances in medicine, 16th edn. Churchill Livingstone, Edinburgh and London

Kerr, D N S, Davidson J M 1975 The assessment of renal function. British Journal of Hospital Medicine 14: 360

Lever A F 1965 The vasa recta and countercurrent multiplication. Acta medica scandinavica 178: suppl. 434: 1

Muehrcke R C 1969 Acute renal failure: diagnosis and management. C V Mosby, St Louis

Ogg C 1970 Chronic renal failure. British Medical Journal iv: 223

Peart W S 1977 The kidney as an endocrine organ. Lancet ii: 543

Pincherle G 1979 Kidney transplants and dialysis. HMSO, London

Robinson J R 1967 Fundamentals of acid-base regulation, 3rd edn. Blackwell, Oxford

Robson J S 1968 Current concepts of renal physiology. Practitioner 201: 413

Wills M R 1971 The biochemical consequences of chronic renal failure. Harvey Miller & Medcalf, Aylesbury, Bucks

8

Jaundice and hepatic failure

One of the most obvious signs of defective hepatic function is jaundice—a yellow discoloration of the skin and sclerae from the accumulation of the bile pigment bilirubin. However, the liver has many functions other than the excretion of haemoglobin breakdown products, and the manifestations of hepatic failure are in consequence protean. Moreover, jaundice may occur from causes other than defective hepatic function, for example, excessive red cell breakdown (haemolytic jaundice), and biliary obstruction outwith the liver (obstructive jaundice).

For this reason the present section is divided into separate discussions of the pathogenesis of jaundice and of hepatic failure.

JAUNDICE

Jaundice occurs when the body is unable to excrete bilirubin as rapidly as it is formed. Thus it occurs both when the rate of bilirubin formation is increased, as in haemolytic anaemia, and when the rate of bilirubin formation is normal but its rate of excretion is reduced, as in hepatic disease and biliary obstruction. Jaundice appears clinically when the concentration of bilirubin in the plasma exceeds about 35 μmol/1 (2 mg/100 ml); the tissues of a patient recovering from jaundice may, however, remain discoloured for some time after the plasma bilirubin concentration has returned to normal.

PHYSIOLOGY

Bilirubin formation
Bilirubin is formed within the cells of the reticuloendothelial system from the haemoglobin of effete red cells. A small amount is formed also in the liver from the breakdown of compounds other than haemoglobin; and some results from the breakdown of immature red cells in the bone marrow. 80 to 85 per cent, however, arises from the

breakdown of aged red cells, which have been ingested by phagocytes in the liver, spleen and bone marrow.

The first step in the breakdown of haemoglobin is the splitting of the molecule into the iron-containing pigment, haem, and the protein moiety, globin. The amino acids which compose the latter enter the body's amino acid pool, where they are available for resynthesis into other proteins, including further globin. Iron, removed from the haem part of the molecule, is transported to the bone marrow attached to the protein, transferrin (see section on anaemia), and reused for the formation of fresh erythrocytes.

The part of the haem molecule which does not contain iron is called protoporphyrin. This compound is converted enzymatically into bilirubin, which is then carried round the body bound to plasma albumin. In this form, bilirubin is relatively insoluble and does not readily cross capillary membranes, for example those of the renal glomeruli and the 'blood-brain barrier'. Plasma-bound bilirubin does not give a 'direct' van den Bergh reaction (see later).

Certain drugs, such as salicylates and sulphonamides, compete for the sites of plasma albumin which bind bilirubin; and, if these drugs are given to jaundiced infants, bilirubin may be displaced from the plasma proteins, so that it can penetrate the blood-brain barrier with serious consequences on the c.n.s. (the condition of kernicterus).

Bilirubin bound to plasma albumin is not filtered in the renal glomeruli, and is therefore not excreted in the urine. Bile-staining of the urine is not a feature of jaundice resulting from excessive haemolysis (acholuric jaundice), because the excess bilirubin has not passed through the hepatic cells and is therefore still in its unconjugated, protein-bound form. (The urine in this condition may, however, be pigmented from the presence of excessive amounts of urobilinogen—see later.)

Bilirubin excretion
Bilirubin is normally removed from the blood by the liver, becoming in the process conjugated with glucuronic acid and thus water-soluble and able to pass through the renal glomerular capilliary membrane. The first step in this process is the active transfer of bilirubin from the plasma into the hepatic cells; congenital absence of the enzyme responsible for this process gives rise to Gilbert's syndrome—a mild form of congenital jaundice. Once inside the hepatic cells, bilirubin becomes conjugated with glucuronic acid under the influence of the enzyme glucuronyl transferase; it is then secreted into the bile canaliculi, and thence into the lumen of the gastrointestinal tract.

Congenital absence of glucuronyl transferase causes a severe form of congenital jaundice—the Crigler-Najjar syndrome. Defective transfer of bilirubin from the hepatic cells into the bile canaliculi gives rise to the relatively benign Dubin-Johnson and Rotor syndromes. Neonates have a mild glucuronyl transferase deficiency, which is probably the chief cause of the physiological jaundice which occurs during the first few days of life. This deficiency is particularly severe in premature infants.

In the lower gut, bilirubin is converted by bacterial action into urobilinogen, which, after oxidation to urobilin (stercobilin), is responsible for the normal dark colour of the faeces. Some urobilinogen is reabsorbed from the lower ileum, and re-excreted by the liver (enterohepatic circulation); a small amount is removed from the blood by the kidneys, and (after oxidization to urobilin) is responsible for the normal yellow colour of the urine.

TYPES OF JAUNDICE

Jaundice may arise in three main ways:

1. Excessive haemolysis, as considered in the section on haemolytic anaemia (q.v.).
2. Intrahepatic hindrance to the transport of bilirubin from the plasma into the small biliary canaliculi, as occurs in the inborn enzymatic defects mentioned above, and in parenchymatous liver disease, such as hepatic necrosis and infective hepatitis. In these conditions there is usually an element of intrahepatic cholestasis, a phenomenon seen also in jaundice from the toxic action of certain drugs, e.g. chlorpromazine.
3. Obstruction of the large extrahepatic biliary channels, e.g. by gallstones, stricture of the common bile duct, or carcinoma of the head of the pancreas.

Jaundice may thus be haemolytic, parenchymatous or obstructive, although in the second condition there is often also an element of intrahepatic obstruction from blockage of intrahepatic bile canaliculi.

CLINICAL FEATURES OF JAUNDICE

Haemolytic jaundice

The etiology of abnormal haemolysis is considered in detail in the section on haemolytic anaemia (q.v.). If the reduction of red cell survival time is not too great, the body may be able to increase its rate of red cell formation sufficiently to keep pace with the increased destruction, so that the peripheral haemoglobin concentration remains within normal limits. If the reduction of red cell survival time is more severe, however, it may be sufficient to cause a reduced haemoglobin concentration—haemolytic anaemia.

When there is increased red cell production the proportion of young red cells (reticulocytes) in the peripheral blood is increased above the normal one or two per cent, and may be as high as 20 or 30 per cent. And in chronic haemolytic anaemia, the red bone marrow may be considerably expanded, and therefore no longer confined, as it normally is, to a small part of the skeleton.

The plasma bilirubin concentration is increased in haemolytic jaundice, although it does not usually exceed about 70 μmol/l (4 mg/100 ml) cf. the very high concentrations found in obstructive jaundice. For reasons considered earlier, the plasma in haemolytic anaemia does not give a 'direct' van den Bergh reaction (the purple colour formed by the addition of Ehrlich's diazo reagent to the blood). Nor does bilirubin appear in the urine. There is, however, increased bilirubin excretion in the bile, and therefore increased amounts of urobilin in both the urine and faeces. Pigment stones, composed mainly of urobilin, may be formed in the gall bladder.

Parenchymatous jaundice

Jaundice from defective hepatocellular function occurs (rarely) as a result of enzymatic defects (see above) and, much more commonly, from the action of toxic or infective agents on the hepatic cells. Thus it may occur as a result of viral hepatitis, leptospirosis (Weil's disease), or septicaemia, or as a result of poisoning with, for example, chloroform, carbon tetrachloride or phosphorus.

Certain drugs, such as chlorpromazine, para-amino salicylic acid and testosterone are particularly likely to cause jaundice in sensitive patients, although it appears that this is the result mainly of allergic cholangitis, causing obstruction of small intrahepatic bile canaliculi, rather than of impaired hepatocellular function.

The ability of the hepatic cells to conjugate bilirubin with glucuronic acid is usually preserved in parenchymatous jaundice, therefore the excess plasma bilirubin is mainly in the water-soluble, conjugated form; bilirubin thus appears in the urine, which is consequently dark in colour.

Obstructive jaundice

Obstructive jaundice may be intrahepatic (as considered above) or extrahepatic, as when there is obstruction to the extrahepatic biliary pathway. As in parenchymatous jaundice, the plasma bilirubin concentration is raised, mainly by increase in the amount of conjugated bilirubin present. The urine is dark; the faeces, however, are pale because urobilinogen (stercobilinogen) is prevented from entering the intestinal lumen.

The obstruction in this type of jaundice impedes the passage of all biliary contents, bile salts as well as bile pigments. Loss of the emulsifying action of bile salts may impair intestinal digestion and absorption, giving rise to steatorrhoea (q.v.) and impaired absorption of the fat-soluble vitamins, particularly vitamin K. Retention of bile salts may give rise also to troublesome pruritus. And lack of the neutralising action of the alkaline bile in the duodenum sometimes results in peptic ulceration of this region of the small intestine.

The enzyme alkaline phosphatase is normally excreted in the bile; its concentration in the plasma may therefore be considerably elevated in obstructive jaundice, and, to a lesser extent, in hepatocellular disease. A high plasma concentration of this enzyme may, however, be found also in the presence of increased osteoblastic activity, such as accompanies Paget's disease, hyperparathyroidism and metastatic bone disease (see Chapter 11).

In clinical practice, differentiation of parenchymatous from obstructive jaundice is difficult; and diagnostic laparotomy is all too frequent an occurrence. Such diagnostic confusion is not, however, entirely surprising in view of the tendency for parenchymatous hepatic disease to have an element of intrahepatic obstruction and cholestasis (see ealier).

HEPATIC FAILURE
PHYSIOLOGY

In addition to its role in excreting red cell breakdown products, the liver has a variety of other metabolic functions, derangement of which gives rise to clinical and biochemical manifestations of hepatic failure. Broadly speaking, the liver's metabolic activities may be considered under three heads: excretion, synthesis, and detoxication.

Excretion
The role of the liver in the excretion of bile salts and alkaline phosphatase has already been considered in the section on obstructive jaundice (q.v.).

Synthesis
The liver is responsible for synthesis of most of the plasma proteins;

the immunoglobulins, however, are formed in reticuloendothelial cells outside the liver. Albumin production is normally at the rate of 10 to 12 g per day. The liver also produces: prothrombin, fibrinogen and most of the other clotting factors (see section on haemorrhagic disorders), the α_2-globulin angiotensinogen (see section on hypertension), and the plasma proteins which carry cortisol (transcortin—see Chapter 10), oestrogens, iron (transferrin—see section on anaemia), and copper (caeruloplasmin).

The liver also plays an important role in carbohydrate and fat metabolism. In the post-absorptive state it converts part of the absorbed glucose into glycogen, which can then be reconverted into glucose as carbohydrate absorption declines. The liver thus plays a major role in minimizing changes in blood glucose concentration between meals. It is also able to synthesize glucose from non-carbohydrate sources, such as amino acids, glycerol and lactic acid (gluconeogenesis); and is a major site for the synthesis of fat from glycerol and free fatty acids.

Detoxication

The liver is concerned with the detoxication of a variety of metabolites and drugs. It converts ammonia, formed by amino acid metabolism, into urea; it also conjugates various steroid hormones, e.g. cortisol (see Chapter 10), oestrogens and testosterone, and their metabolites, thus rendering them water-soluble and liable (after enterohepatic circulation) to renal excretion.

The role of the liver in the metabolism of drugs such as opiates, barbiturates and steroid hormones, is particularly important; these substances should be administered with care to patients who have impaired hepatic function. The regular administration of barbiturates increases the activity of hepatic microsomal enzymes, and thus increases the liver's ability to detoxicate other drugs, such as steroid hormones and anticoagulants. This phenomenon is known as enzyme induction and is now recognized as being a major source of interaction between a variety of commonly-used drugs (see standard texts on pharmacology).

Haemodynamics

The liver receives a dual blood supply from the hepatic artery and portal vein. The total blood flow is in the region of 1½ l/min; in the normal liver about one-quarter of this comes from the hepatic artery. It has been estimated that some 70 per cent of the liver's oxygen supply comes via the portal vein, which, of course, contains partially deoxygenated blood from the gastrointestinal tract. The hydrostatic pressure in the portal vein is low, normally in the region of 6 to 12 mmHg (0.8 to 1.6 kPa) in hepatic disease, however, it may become considerably raised—the condition of portal hypertension (see later).

PATHOGENESIS OF HEPATIC FAILURE

Hepatic failure arises usually as the end-result of a progressive deterioration of hepatic function from some chronic pathological process. Rarely, however, the condition may be acute, as when the hepatic cells are damaged by chemical poisons such as carbon tetra-chloride, or by an overwhelming infection, as by the virus of infective hepatitis.

Fortunately, the liver has a large functional reserve; and a pathological process must be extensive before it can cause the manifestations of hepatic failure. A sudden, large increase of metabolic load may, however, be sufficient to induce hepatic failure in a patient with a previously well-compensated defect of hepatic function. The commonest example of such acute-on-chronic failure is that which sometimes follows gastrointestinal haemorrhage in a cirrhotic patient. (A large gastrointestinal bleed is equivalent to a large protein meal, and therefore represents a severe stress on the liver's impaired metabolic ability.)

Cirrhosis
The commonest cause of chronic hepatic failure is cirrhosis of the liver. A detailed discussion of the etiology of this condition would be out of place here; the various possible causative mechanisms will, however, be briefly considered.

The essential pathology of cirrhosis is destruction of the normal hepatic architecture, and replacement of hepatic cells by over-growth of fibrous tissue. This may occur as the end-result of a variety of pathological processes.

The most usual type of cirrhosis is portal, or Laennec's, cirrhosis. This may be a late consequence of the acute necrosis of a large area of liver; or, more commonly, the result of the chronic action of some less virulent pathological process.

Undoubtedly, an excessive intake of alcohol over a prolonged period of time is an important etiological factor in portal cirrhosis; 50 per cent of cirrhotics are alcoholics, and 10 per cent of alcoholics have cirrhosis. A recent survey has shown that in London as many as 65 per cent of cases with diagnosed cirrhosis have alcohol as a major etiological factor; and in some parts of the world the figure may be as high as 90 per cent. This relationship between excessive alcohol intake and cirrhosis is also indicated by the fact that publicans are some seven times more likely to die from cirrhosis than people in other employment. It is not clear, however, what is the relative importance of excessive alcohol intake *per se* and the defective general nutrition which accompanies chronic alcoholism. A similar picture may occur in chronic malnutrition in the absence of alcoholism.

Rarely, this condition may occur as a result of a metabolic disorder. In haemochromatosis, intestinal iron absorption is excessive, so that the plasma iron concentration is increased; as a result, iron is deposited in certain organs, particularly the liver, pancreas, heart and skin. In the liver it causes fibrosis and cirrhosis. (The other manifestations of this condition include diabetes mellitus, cardiomyopathy, and a characteristic bronze discoloration of the skin, which accounts for its synonym—'bronzed diabetes'.) In Wilson's disease there is deficiency of the copper-carrying plasma protein, caeruloplasmin; copper is therefore deposited in the liver, the basal ganglia of the brain and the cornea. In the liver this results in cirrhosis.

Biliary cirrhosis arises as a result of intrahepatic or extrahepatic obstruction of the biliary tracts. This is especially the case when obstruction is associated with ascending biliary infection—ascending cholangitis. Cardiac cirrhosis is a result of the chronic venous congestion which accompanies congestive cardiac failure (q.v.).

CLINICAL FEATURES OF HEPATIC FAILURE

In accord with the liver's multiplicity of functions, the clinical manifestations of hepatic failure are widespread. The liver has, however, a large functional reserve and considerable regenerative powers. Damage must therefore be extensive before it can give rise to clinical manifestations of hepatic failure. Also, some hepatic functions, particularly those concerned with carbohydrate metabolism, may be taken over by other organs, the function of which is not impaired in hepatic failure.

Jaundice
In view of the liver's obvious role in bile pigment metabolism, it might be thought that one of the most obvious manifestations of hepatic failure would be jaundice. In fact, however, severe jaundice is not usually a feature of this condition, except when it is due to acute hepatic damage, e.g. a fulminating attack of viral hepatitis.

The jaundice of hepatic failure is due mainly to impaired hepatocellular function. This takes the form of decreased bilirubin uptake by the hepatic cells, and failure of bilirubin conjugation within the cells.

There is usually also an element of intrahepatic cholestasis. In chronic hepatic failure erythrocyte survival time may be considerably reduced; jaundice is then aggravated by haemolysis.

Impaired synthesis of proteins, fats and carbohydrates

In acute hepatic failure there may be hypoglycaemia as a result of the liver's inability to produce glucose from non-carbohydrate sources; and a reduction in blood urea concentration from its inability to deaminate amino acids. In chronic failure glucose uptake by the hepatic cells may be impaired, so that the patient's glucose tolerance curve resembles that seen in diabetes mellitus (q.v.), with a high peak and a slow decay (see Fig. 18).

Protein synthesis is also markedly abnormal. Thus, there is generalized muscular wasting and hypoalbuminaemia (a contributory cause to the oedema which commonly accompanies hepatic failure—see later). And since the liver is unable to metabolize amino acids such as methionine and cystine, these are present in the urine in excessive amounts (aminoaciduria). Gamma-globulin synthesis is not impaired, because this occurs mainly outside the liver, in the cells of the reticuloendothelial system.

Defective formation of various clotting factors (chiefly prothrombin and factor VII) may cause an abnormal bleeding tendency. This may be aggravated by platelet deficiency from the splenomegaly (hypersplenism) which accompanies portal hypertension (see below).

The liver is normally responsible for cholesterol esterification, therefore in hepatic failure the ratio of esterified to unesterified cholesterol is often decreased. In obstructive jaundice there is an increase in the plasma cholesterol concentration, due mainly to the fact that cholesterol is not being converted into bile salts.

Failure to catabolize certain hormones and toxic metabolites

Hepatic failure impairs the ability of the liver to metabolize certain hormones, and is thus commonly associated with symptoms of hormonal overactivity. Thus the plasma aldosterone concentration may be raised, leading to sodium retention and expansion of the extracellular fluid (see section on sodium balance); there may also be defective metabolism of ADH, causing water retention. (As a result of the low plasma albumin concentration commonly found in hepatic failure, excess extracellular fluid tends to accumulate in the interstitial fluid compartment, causing oedema.)

Excessive extracellular fluid tends to accumulate also within the peritoneal cavity, causing ascites. The preferential accumulation of fluid in this situation seems to be due mainly to increased capillary pressure, secondary to portal hypertension (see below), and perhaps also to lymphatic obstruction within the liver.

In the male, impaired oestrogen metabolism results in feminization, with gynaecomastia and testicular atrophy; and, in both sexes, in palmar erythema ('liver palms') and cutaneous vascular abnormalities (spider naevi). It should be stressed that the correlation between the presence of such clinical manifestations of hyperoestrogenism and biochemical evidence of impaired oestrogen metabolism is poor.

The low grade fever which may accompany chronic hepatic failure may be due to inability to detoxicate some (unknown) pyrogen, perhaps some substance absorbed from the gut. It may also be associated with the fact that, in this condition, Gram negative intestinal bacteria are able to bypass the liver through portasystemic anastomoses. (For this reason also septic shock is particularly common in cirrhotic patients—see p. 19).

The metabolism of certain drugs, e.g. morphine, may be severely impaired in patients with hepatic failure.

Hyperdynamic circulation

Patients with chronic hepatic failure often have an above-normal cardiac output, and a decreased systemic total peripheral resistance (see section on hypertension). There are several reasons for this hyperdynamic circulation: blood volume is increased by excess aldosterone and ADH activity (see above); the patient may be anaemic, so that the oxygen-carrying capacity of his peripheral blood is reduced; and it is thought that an abnormal vasodilator substance may be present in the peripheral blood. As a result of the first two factors, cardiac output is increased (see sections on peripheral circulatory failure and anaemia, respectively); this increase is, however, accompanied by a reduction of total peripheral resistance, so the systemic arterial pressure is not raised (see section on hypertension).

Increase of cardiac output in hepatic failure is accompanied by a decrease of myocardial and renal blood flow. There is thus a redistribution of blood flow towards the extremities, which are, in consequence, warm and show capillary pulsation.

There is also marked vasodilation in the pulmonary circulation, probably the result of the opening up of arteriovenous fistulae, with consequent right-to-left intrapulmonary shunting and arterial hypoxaemia (see section on respiratory failure).

Ascites

The accumulation of fluid within the peritoneal cavity (ascites), which accompanies hepatic cirrhosis has been mentioned already. It is the result of several factors; and the relative importance of hypoalbuminaemia, sodium and water retention, and increased portal venous pressure probably vary from patient to patient. Unlike the fluid which accumulates in infective and neoplastic conditions, ascitic fluid is relatively protein-free, a fact of diagnostic importance.

In addition to ascites, cirrhotic patients may develop pleural effusions.

Portal hypertension

Hepatic fibrosis tends to impede blood flow through the liver, so that portal venous pressure is considerably above normal—the condition of portal hypertension. This is usually associated with the presence of abnormal communications between the portal and systemic veins, particularly those around the lower end of the oesophagus, in the wall of the rectum, and around the umbilicus (*caput medusae*). Such oesophageal varices are particularly prone to haemorrhage, which may precipitate hepatic coma (see below). In addition, bypass channels may open up in the liver and allow portal venous blood to transverse this organ without coming into contact with functioning hepatic cells.

Hypersplenism

Portal hypertension is usually accompanied by chronic splenic engorgement and splenomegaly. This may result in 'hypersplenism', a condition in which the formed elements of the blood are destroyed abnormally rapidly by excessive reticuloendothelial activity in the enlarged spleen. The resulting thrombocytopenia (q.v.) may aggravate an already-present haemorrhagic tendency from defective formation of clotting factors.

Portasystemic encephalopathy and neuropsychiatric manifestations of hepatic failure

Certain forms of hepatic failure are associated with marked neurological and psychiatric manifestations. These appear to be due mainly to the action of various (unknown) substances which the damaged liver is unable to detoxicate, either because its functioning cells are bypassed by portasystemic anastomoses, or because their metabolic activity is severely depressed.

One of the putative toxins is ammonia, although other substances are almost certainly involved. The concentration of ammonia in the blood is particularly likely to be raised when the patient is on a high-protein diet; and the large protein load represented by a severe gastrointestinal haemorrhage (due commonly to a ruptured oesophageal varix) may be sufficient to precipitate a patient with defective hepatic function into coma. Such coma may be reversed by purgation, and by the administration of antibiotics which reduce ammonia production by bacterial action within the intestinal lumen.

The most common psychiatric manifestations of hepatic failure are personality changes and intellectual impairment; in severe cases, the patient may become comatose (hepatic coma). In addition, there may be neurological signs, such as hyperreflexia and the characteristic (but not pathognomonic) flapping tremor of the outstretched hands. In late cases there may be irreversible c.n.s. damage, with paraplegia and dementia.

Hepatic foetor

The breath of patients with hepatic failure commonly has a characteristic musty odour (hepatic foetor), the intensity of which correlates with the severity of their neuropsychiatric manifestations (see above), and which is due presumably to the same toxic metabolites.

FURTHER READING

Anon 1977 Fulminant hepatic failure. British Medical Journal ii: 1301
Anon 1978 Hereditary jaundice. Lancet ii: 926
Campbell E J M, Dickinson C J, Slater J D H 1974 Clinical physiology, 4th edn. Blackwell, Oxford, ch 13
Heathcote E J L 1977 Hepatitis. In: Baron D N, Compston N, Dawson A M (ed) Recent advances in medicine, 17th edn. Churchill Livingstone, Edinburgh and London
Heaton K W 1977 Alcohol and liver disease. British Journal of Hospital Medicine 18: 118
Hoffman W S 1970 The biochemistry of clinical medicine, 4th edn. Year Book Medical Publishers, Chicago, ch 9
Losowsky M S, Scott B B 1973 Hepatic encephalopathy. British Medical Journal iii: 279
McIntyre N 1975 Cirrhosis of the liver. British Journal of Hospital Medicine 13: 8
Paton A 1968 Jaundice. British Medical Journal i: 164
Read A E 1968 Cirrhosis of the liver. British Medical Journal i: 427
Richards J D M 1976 Hypersplenism. British Journal of Hospital Medicine 15: 505
Sherlock S 1968 Drugs and the liver. British Medical Journal i: 227
Sherlock S 1973 Acute virus hepatitis. Practitioner 210: 603
Sherlock S 1975 Diseases of the liver and biliary system, 5th edn. Blackwell, Oxford
Sherlock S 1977 Hepatic encephalopathy. British Journal of Hospital Medicine 17: 144
Stone W D 1973 Cirrhosis of the liver. Practitioner 210: 612
Thompson R P H 1970 Recent advances in jaundice: physiology. British Medical Journal i: 223

9

The malabsorption syndrome

The function of the gastrointestinal tract is to break down complex dietary foodstuffs (fats, carbohydrates, proteins, etc.) into simpler molecules and then to absorb these breakdown products into the body, where they can enter its various metabolic pathways. Malabsorption occurs when the gastrointestinal tract fails to carry out its normal function adequately; clearly, this situation may arise either because the digestive processes are incomplete, or because the absorptive processes are impaired, or because both aspects of gastrointestinal function are deranged simultaneously.

The manifestations of malabsorption—the malabsorption syndrome—depend partly on whether the cause is a relatively specific enzyme defect, e.g. disaccharidase deficiency, or whether there is a general loss of gastrointestinal function, such as occurs in gluten-sensitive enteropathy. They depend also on the patient's pre-existing physiological and biochemical weaknesses; one patient may complain chiefly of diarrhoea, another may be severely anaemic, another may present with skeletal demineralization, and yet another may have a complex symptomatology from multiple biochemical deficiencies.

PHYSIOLOGY

The majority of the gastrointestinal digestive processes occur in the small intestine; salivary amylase and the gastric enzymes are not essential to normal health.*

Carbohydrates

The chief enzymes concerned with the digestion of dietary carbohydrates are pancreatic amylase and the disaccharidases (lactase, maltase, isomaltase and invertase) which are found in the brush borders of the cells which line the intestinal villi. The enzymes of the so-called 'succus entericus' are now thought to be derived by desquamation of lining cells into the intestinal lumen.

*Lack of intrinsic factor, however, as after a total gastrectomy, in time causes severe anaemia (see Chapter 5).

Pancreatic secretion is controlled partly by the vagus and partly by the hormones secretin and pancreozymin, which are liberated from the duodenal mucosa in response to the presence there of gastric chyme. Secretin controls mainly the electrolyte composition of the pancreatic juice, pancreozymin controls its enzymatic content.

Pancreatic amylase breaks down dietary polysaccharides, such as starch, into simpler disaccharides, such as maltose and isomaltose. These disaccharides, together with others (such as lactose) which are ingested as such, are then broken down into their constituent monosaccharides—glucose, galactose, fructose, etc.—within the cells lining the intestinal villi. Monosaccharides liberated in this way are then transferred into capillary networks inside the villi. Transfer of glucose and galactose is an active process which requires the expenditure of metabolically-produced energy, and is thus capable of propelling these substances against chemical concentration gradients; the absorption of other sugars, such as fructose, is purely passive.

Fats

The chief enzyme concerned with fat digestion is pancreatic lipase. The action of this enzyme is to break down triglycerides into di- and monoglycerides and free fatty acids. In this action it is considerably aided by the emulsifying action of bile salts, discharged into the duodenum under the influence of the intestinal hormone, 'cholecystokinin', which is now thought to be identical to pancreozymin. Bile is concerned also with emulsifying the products of fat digestion which are themselves but sparingly water-soluble. The resulting fine emulsion of monoglycerides and long-chain fatty acids is absorbed into the cells which line the intestinal villi. Here the products of digestion recombine to form triglycerides, which then pass to lymphatics (lacteals) in the centres of the villi.

Vitamins A, D, E and K are absorbed in conjunction with the finally-divided emulsion of fat breakdown products just considered. Anything which impedes fat absorption may cause deficiencies of these fat-soluble vitamins.

Proteins

Digestion of dietary proteins occurs mainly under the control of the pancreatic enzymes, trypsin, chymotrypsin and carboxypeptidase. These enzymes are secreted in an inactive (zymogen) form, which only becomes active in the duodenum on contact with enterokinase or with already-formed trypsin. Aided to some extent by gastric pepsin, these pancreatic enzymes digest proteins to peptides which are then taken up into the cells lining the intestinal villi. Here the process of digestion to amino acids is completed by peptidases present in the brush borders of the villous lining cells.

The amino acids so formed are then actively transported into the mucosal capillaries. There appear to be at least two separate enzyme systems which are concerned with the transport of amino acids: one system transports cystine and dibasic amino acids, the other transports neutral amino acids.

Minerals

From the point of view of the malabsorption syndrome the most important minerals are iron and calcium. Iron is liberated from combination with organic materials by gastric hydrochloric acid, and is then actively absorbed (in the ferrous form) from the jejunum and upper ileum. Iron absorption is adjusted in accordance with the body's needs by the degree of saturation or otherwise of the mucosal protein, apoferritin. When the body is depleted of iron this protein is in the non-iron containing form so that iron absorption occurs readily; but when the body's iron stores are full the mucosal protein is mainly combined with iron (that is in the form of ferritin) and therefore unavailable to aid further iron absorption. (Overabsorption of iron results in the condition of haemochromatosis—see section on hepatic failure—in which excessive amounts of iron-containing pigments are deposited in the liver and pancreas, with deleterious consequences to the function of these organs. This condition may occur as a result of frequent blood transfusions, or of a congenital deficiency of the mechanism which normally limits intestinal iron absorption.)

The absorption of calcium requires the presence in the body of an adequate amount of vitamin D; it is also, to some extent, under the control of parathyroid hormone (see Chapter 10). Calcium absorption is impaired by anthing which prevents the absorption of fats from the small intestine, because unabsorbed fatty acids combine with calcium to form insoluble calcium soaps, which are not absorbed. Malabsorption, particularly of fats, may also cause deficiency of the fat-soluble vitamin D, and a secondary impairment of calcium absorption.

There is a gradient of absorptive activity down the small intestine from the jejunum to the terminal ileum. The absorptive capacity of the intestine is greatest in the jejunum, and it is here also that the greatest amount of substrate is available for absorption. The small intestine has a large functional reserve, and much of this organ may be removed surgically without causing a noticeable impairment of absorptive ability.

PATHOGENESIS OF MALABSORPTION SYNDROME

Failure of digestion

The commonest causes of malabsorption within this category are deficient secretion of pancreatic enzymes as a result of, for example, chronic pancreatitis, and deficient secretion of bile salts, such as occurs in obstructive jaundice (q.v.). Deficient secretion of bile salts may occur also in hepatocellular disease (q.v.), and when the entero-hepatic circulation of these salts is impaired by lesions of the terminal ileum, where the majority of bile salt reabsorption normally occurs.

Digestion may be impaired also when the pancreatic enzymes and bile fail to meet their substrates in the duodenal lumen. This may happen, for example, in patients with a gastrojejunostomy, when the gastric contents may pass straight into the jejunum without mixing with the duodenal digestive juices. Digestion may then be impaired further by the fact that the hormones which normally stimulate pancreatic and biliary secretion, and which are normally liberated by contact of food with the duodenal mucosa, are released only in reduced amounts.

Digestion is impaired also in disaccharidase deficiency (see next section).

Failure of absorption

Reduction of absorptive surface area

An obvious cause of malabsorption is reduction of the absorptive area of the intestinal mucosa as a result of surgical resection. There is normally, however, a large reserve of mucosal function, and malabsorption tends not to occur until a large proportion of the small intestine has been resected. An exception is the absorption of vitamin B_{12}; this is absorbed mainly from the terminal few feet of ileum, therefore resection of this part of the gut, as for Crohn's disease, may cause vitamin B_{12} deficiency and a megaloblastic anaemia (q.v.).

Damage to the intestinal mucosa

The commonest cause of malabsorption within this category is gluten-sensitive enteropathy, which manifests itself as coeliac disease in children and as idiopathic steatorrhoea in adults. In this condition the small intestine is sensitive in some way to the gluten component of cereals in the diet, with the result that the mucosa is damaged and unable adequately to absorb various substances, particularly fats. The cause of this mucosal damage is uncertain: it may be an immunological sensitivity reaction, or it may be due to lack of a specific mucosal enzyme which normally breaks down some otherwise toxic product of gluten digestion.

Damage to the intestinal mucosa and malabsorption may occur also when the mucosa is infiltrated by a reticulosis, or by a granulomatous process such as Crohn's disease, or by an infiltration of unknown origin, as occurs in Whipple's disease.

In disaccharidase deficiency there is a defect of the mucosal disaccharidases, with the result that the appropriate disaccharide (commonly lactose) cannot be adequately absorbed. This condition occurs either as an inborn error of metabolism, when there is an isolated enzyme defect, or as the result of generalized mucosal damage, as in gluten-sensitive enteropathy.

Impaired intestinal blood or lymph flow

Malabsorption may occur because the flow of blood or of lymph through the absorptive area of the intestine is reduced, for example by mesenteric arterial insufficiency or malignant infiltration of the intestinal lymphatics. The former condition may give rise to 'abdominal angina' which is rather analogous to angina pectoris and intermittent claudication. In this condition the increased metabolic demands which accompany digestion produce abdominal pain, coming on soon after a meal, and then waning as the digestive process is completed.

Products of digestion metabolized or otherwise altered by intestinal bacteria, etc.

Infestation of the small intestine with the fish tapeworm *Diphyllobothrium latum* causes malabsorption of vitamin B_{12}, because the worm takes for its own use the B_{12} which would normally be absorbed into the body. Vitamin B_{12} deficiency from this cause is, however, excessively rare.

Proliferation of bacteria in blind loops of small intestine, in diverticula, or in dilated bowel proximal to an intestinal stricture may also cause symptoms of malabsorption. It appears that, in this 'blind loop syndrome', the bile salts which are necessary for efficient digestion and absorption (see earlier) are split by bacterial action, thus causing impaired fat absorption and steatorrhoea. It has also been suggested that certain products of bile salt metabolism may be toxic to the intestinal mucosa, and may thus cause an impairment of gastrointestinal function. The clinical state of patients with the 'blind loop syndrome' may often be dramatically improved by small doses of oral antibiotics.

MANIFESTATIONS OF MALABSORPTION

The manifestations of malabsorption vary widely from patient to patient, but may be divided into those, such as steatorrhoea and diarrhoea, which are due primarily to the presence of various unabsorbed substances in the intestine, and into signs and symptoms which are the result of deficiencies of various essential nutrients. In this latter category may be included: deficiencies of iron, folic acid and vitamin B_{12} causing anaemia (q.v.), of calcium causing tetany and osteomalacia (q.v.), and of vitamin K causing a haemorrhagic tendency due to deficiency of several clotting factors (chiefly factor VII)—see Chapter 6.

Patients with severe malabsorption usually have steatorrhoea (see below); but this is not inevitable, and a patient with gross multiple deficiencies from malabsorption may have stools which are macroscopically, and even biochemically, normal. Steatorrhoea is by no means synonymous with malabsorption.

Diarrhoea and steatorrhoea
These symptoms occur mainly in the more severe forms of the syndrome. Patients with gross steatorrhoea have stools which contain excessive amounts of fat, and these therefore tend to be pale, bulky, greasy and to float on water. In less severe cases the patient's stools may be macroscopically normal, although on biochemical analysis they contain abnormal amounts of fat. The normal laboratory test for steatorrhoea is to collect the faeces for three days while the patient is on a normal mixed diet, and then to determine their fat content. An average faecal fat loss of more than 6 g/24 hours is diagnostic of steatorrhoea.

Abdominal distension, colic, etc.
A prominent feature of the malabsorption syndrome is abdominal distension, due either to the presence of excessive intestinal gas from bacterial fermentation of unabsorbed carbohydrates or fatty acids, or to the presence of an excessive amount of fluid in the intestinal lumen. Such distension may be accompanied by colicky abdominal pain, which is occasionally so severe as to suggest intestinal obstruction. The marked abdominal distension is in sharp contrast to the wasting of the rest of the body which occurs in the severer forms of the condition (see below).

Anaemia
Anaemia as a result of malabsorption may be microcytic and hypo-

chromic when due to iron deficiency, or megaloblastic when due to deficiency of vitamin B_{12} or folic acid (see Chapter 5). Iron deficiency may be accompanied by manifestations of the Plummer-Vinson syndrome—glossitis, koilonychia and dysphagia; deficiency of vitamin B_{12} may cause subacute combined degeneration of the spinal cord, as it does in Addisonian pernicious anaemia.

A combination of deficiencies may produce a mixed blood picture, in which the anaemia is both macrocytic (m.c.v. > 94 fl) and hypochromic (m.c.h.c. < 32 g/dl). Even when one type of anaemia is dominant, relief of the major deficiency may reveal a subclinical deficiency of some other essential factor.

Vitamin deficiencies

Except for deficiency of vitamin B_{12} (see above), the deficiencies which occur in this category are mainly those of the fat-soluble vitamins. Clinically, the most important deficiencies are those of vitamins D and K.

Deficiency of vitamin D is partially responsible for the defective calcium absorption which may occur in patients with various forms of malabsorption. (The other cause is the combination of calcium with unabsorbed fatty acids to form insoluble calcium soaps—see earlier.) The consequences of such defective absorption are considered below.

Deficiency of vitamin K gives rise to a haemorrhagic tendency, due primarily to deficiency of factor VII; there is also defective production of factor II (prothrombin) and of factors IX and X. Deficiency of these various factors results in a variety of haemorrhagic manifestations, including purpura and gastrointestinal bleeding (see Chapter 6).

Calcium deficiency and skeletal abnormalities

Defective calcium absorption gives rise to a low plasma calcium concentration, and neuromuscular hyperexcitability, with tetany, or latent tetany, as shown by a positive Chvostek's or Trousseau's sign. In some patients the low plasma calcium concentration induces increased secretion of parathyroid hormone, with consequent increased resorption of calcium from the bones, and osteomalacia accompanied by increased plasma alkaline phosphatase activity (see Chapter 11).

The severe protein deficiency which may occur in the malabsorption syndrome (see below) sometimes causes osteoporosis with crush fractures of the vertebrae and other skeletal abnormalities.

Hypoproteinaemia

In addition to having defective protein absorption due directly to their intestinal abnormality, patients with the malabsorption syndrome often feel generally unwell, and poor appetite leads to poor protein intake. In some patients protein deficiency due to reduced intake and defective absorption is aggravated by additional protein loss into the lumen of the gut—protein-losing enteropathy.

Patients with severe malabsorption may therefore exhibit signs of protein deficiency and, except for their protuberant abdomens, appear generally emaciated, with peripheral oedema from hypoalbuminaemia (see section on oedema).

Miscellaneous manifestations

Poor energy (caloric) intake leads to lethargy and weakness. These symptoms may be aggravated by hypokalaemia, occurring as a result of excessive potassium loss from the gut. Some patients complain of sore mouths due to vitamin deficiency, particularly deficiency of various members of the B group. The glossitis of the Plummer-Vinson syndrome has already been mentioned. Vitamin deficiency may account also for the peripheral neuropathy shown by some patients, although this condition is not always relieved by vitamin supplements, suggesting that there is an additional, unknown factor involved in its causation.

Some patients have skin lesions, such as eczema, which are thought to be due partly to vitamin deficiency and partly to unknown causes. Cutaneous pigmentation may be a marked feature; and this, combined with the lethargy shown by these patients, may wrongly suggest a diagnosis of adrenal cortical failure (Addison's disease—q.v.). Rarely, patients with the malabsorption syndrome have clubbing of the fingers and a low grade fever.

PHYSIOLOGICAL PRINCIPLES OF TREATMENT

As with other conditions, specific treatment should be used if available; otherwise attempts should be made to reverse the patient's various biochemical abnormalities by dietary and pharmacological means. In the category of specific treatment are the elimination of lactose (milk, etc.) from the diet of patients with primary or secondary disaccharidase deficiency, and the giving of a gluten-free diet to patients with gluten-sensitive enteropathy. Patients with defective pancreatic function may be improved by the oral administration of preparations containing pancreatic enzymes (pancreatin).

In the absence of specific therapy, treatment must be symptomatic only. The diet should have a low fat content (to prevent steatorrhoea and diarrhoea from intestinal fermentation of fatty acids), but should contain large amounts of protein and carbohydrates to correct hypoalbuminaemia and deficient energy intake. In addition, the patient should receive supplements of those substances in which he is most likely to be deficient, i.e. the fat-soluble vitamins D and K, calcium, and iron, folic acid and vitamin B_{12}. Broad spectrum antibiotics may dramatically improve patients with the 'blind loop syndrome'; they also reduce intestinal fermentation, and may have beneficial effects in patients with malabsorption from other causes.

FURTHER READING

Badenoch J 1960 Steatorrhoea in the adult. British Medical Journal ii: 879, 963

Campbell E J M, Dickinson C J, Slater J D H 1974 Clinical physiology, 4th edn. Blackwell, Oxford, ch 12

Cook W T 1976 Common problems of malabsorption. Practitioner 216: 637

Davenport H W 1965 Physiology of the digestive tract, 2nd edn. Year Book Medical Publishers, Chicago

Dawson A M 1968 Disaccharidase deficiency in man. Post-graduate Medical Journal 44: 646

Dyer N H, Dawson A M 1968 Malabsorption. British Medical Journal ii: 161

Greenberger N J, Winship D H 1976 Gastrointestinal disorders: a pathophysiologic approach. Year Book Medical Publishers, Chicago, ch 3

Matthews D M 1968 Intestinal absorption. British Journal of Hospital Medicine 2: 1382

Naish J M, Read A E 1974 Basic gastroenterology, 2nd edn. Wright, Bristol, ch 17

Saunders D R, McDonald G B 1976 Fat absorption. In: Bouchier I A D (ed) Recent advances in gastroenterology, Churchill Livingstone, Edinburgh

Truelove S C, Jewell D P 1973 Topics in gastroenterology. Blackwell, Oxford, ch 9, 10

Wormsley K G 1977 Pancreatic exocrine physiology. British Journal of Hospital Medicine 18: 518

10

Endocrine defects

The first hormone to be discovered, by Bayliss and Starling in 1902, was secretin—a hormone which controls the exocrine secretion of the pancreas. Now every first year student is familiar with the concept of a hormone as being a substance which is produced in one tissue, and is then carried via the blood stream to affect the activity of some other, remote tissue. In recent years this concept has been widened somewhat to include substances such as angiotensin (see section on hypertension) which are not secreted by definitive endocrine organs, but which are formed from precursors within the circulation; and also to include hormones such as the hypothalamic releasing factors which are not secreted into the general circulation, but which act locally via the hypothalamo-hypophyseal portal system (see below).

In recent years, also, quite a lot has been learned about the way in which hormones influence the metabolism of their target organs. There seem to be two main modes of action; the steroid hormones appear to penetrate into the interior of the cells where they combine with specific nuclear receptor sites, thereby influencing gene transcription and protein (including enzyme) synthesis; the polypeptide hormones interact with specific cell-membrane receptors to activate the adenyl cyclase system, thus increasing the intracellular level of cyclic AMP, and thereby activating a variety of intracellular enzymes. Much however remains to be discovered about this rapidly growing aspect of endocrinology.

It used to be said that the pituitary was the 'leader of the endocrine orchestra'. And this is still true, except that it has become clear in recent years that the release of pituitary hormones is itself under the control of the hypothalamus. This region of the brain produces a variety of 'releasing factors' which are secreted into the hypothalamo-hypophyseal portal vessels, and are then carried down the pituitary stalk to affect the release of trophic hormones from the anterior pituitary. These trophic hormones then in turn affect the activity of a variety of peripheral target organs—adrenal, thyroid, gonads, etc.

THYROID

PHYSIOLOGY

The thyroid gland secretes two iodine-containing hormones, thyroxine (tetraiodothyronine, T4) and triiodothyronine (T3). These are produced within the gland from the precursors, mono- and diiodotyrosine. For simplicity T3 and T4 may be referred to together as thyroid hormone (TH). In the peripheral blood thyroxine is in the majority (90 per cent), and both T3 and T4 are carried mainly in the protein-bound form—chiefly on thyroid-binding globulin (TBG), which is normally about 20 per cent saturated. The level of circulating TH may conveniently be assessed by measuring the concentration of protein-bound iodine in the peripheral blood (but see below).

Iodine is necessary for the formation of TH. The main dietary source of this element is fish and iodised salt. Ingested iodine is absorbed from the small intestine, and is then actively taken up into the thyroid gland; this transport mechanism is particularly active when there is thyroid overactivity, or iodine deficiency. It may be blocked by certain drugs, such as thiocyanate or perchlorate ions.

Once inside the gland the iodine is oxidized and incorporated into tyrosine residues of the protein thyroglobulin to form mono- and diiodotyrosine, which then combine to form T3 and T4 (still combined with thyroglobulin). TH is stored in the colloid of the thyroid acini, from where it is released into the bloodstream under the influence of thyroid stimulating hormone (TSH), a trophic hormone secreted by the pituitary. TSH also stimulates other aspects of thyroid function including the synthesis of TH.

The thiouracils, propyl and methyl thiouracil, and carbimazole inhibit the oxidation of iodide to iodine, and also prevent the incorporation of iodine into the amino acid residues of thyroglobulin, thus inhibiting TH synthesis. They are therefore valuable clinically in the treatment of thyroid overactivity.

In clinical hyperthyroidism there appears to be abnormal thyroid stimulation by a large molecular weight globulin (long acting thyroid stimulator, LATS). But the role (if any) which LATS plays in the normal control of thyroid function is uncertain.

The precise mechanism of action of TH at tissue level is uncertain. Reduction in the rate of thyroid secretion is, however, followed by deficient growth and maturation, and by a decrease in the body's basal metabolic rate, as measured by its oxygen consumption and heat production. Excess thyroid secretion is accompanied by an increased metabolic rate, and by a generalized increase in metabolic activity.

Qualitatively, the effects of T3 and thyroxine are indistinguishable;

but the former is much more rapidly acting because it is less firmly bound to plasma protein. Also, weight for weight T3 has considerably greater metabolic activity.

Assessment of thyroid function

The diagnosis of thyroid malfunction is normally made on clinical grounds and then confirmed by a variety of biochemical tests, some of which are discussed briefly below.

The thyroid takes up radioactive iodine with the same avidity as it does non-radioactive iodine, thus providing a valuable means of assessing thyroid function. Two radio isotopes are available: I^{131} with a half-life of 8 days, and I^{132} with a much shorter half-life. The amount of radio-iodine in the thyroid may be measured externally, by measuring the radioactivity over the gland with a scintillation counter. The time course of thyroid radioactivity varies according to the gland's metabolism; in hyperfunction the radioactivity peak is both higher than normal, and occurs earlier; in underactivity it is lower, and occurs later.

But there are fallacies: in renal disease iodine excretion is depressed, therefore thyroid uptake is enhanced even when the rate of TH formation is normal; in iodine deficiency the thyroid gland removes iodine from the blood at an increased rate; and in patients who have taken large amounts of iodine (e.g., certain medicines or iodine-containing X-ray contrast media) thyroid iodine uptake is depressed.

It is also possible in this way to investigate how the thyroid responds to injections of TSH, and thus to see whether a defect of thyroid function is due to thyroid underactivity *per se* or to pituitary disease (see later).

The concentration of protein bound iodine (PBI) in the peripheral blood normally gives a good measurement of the concentration of circulating TH (see earlier). But in conditions such as the nephrotic syndrome and other forms of hypoproteinaemia, in which there is a deficienty of TBG, the PBI may be low even when the concentration of free TH (and therefore peripheral thyroid hormone activity) is normal. Conversely, the PBI may be artifically high when there is an increase in the available TH binding sites, as in pregnancy, or in patients taking steroid contraceptives, or certain other drugs e.g. phenothiazine or clofibrate. Measurement of PBI is now being replaced by direct measurements of thyroid hormones in the blood.

It used to be common practice to measure the patient's metabolic rate under carefully controlled conditions—the basal metabolic rate (BMR), to assess his thyroid function. This is conveniently done by measuring his oxygen consumption with a close-circuit spirometer, and thence calculating his metabolic rate (1 1 oxygen $\simeq$ 4.8 Cal $\simeq$ 20.6 kJ). Although this test has the theoretical advantage that it is the only way to assess the actual peripheral effects of thyroid activity, it is difficult to perform accurately, and has now generally fallen into disuse.

HYPOTHYROIDISM

Hypothyroidism occurs either as a result of pituitary underactivity (q.v.), or much more commonly from deficient activity of the thyroid gland itself. This latter condition may be due to a congenital deficiency of one of the enzymes which are responsible for TH formation, to impairment of thyroid metabolism by iodine deficiency or ingestion of a drug or other substance with antithyroid activity, to extirpation of the gland either by surgery or irradiation, or (most commonly) to an autoimmunine process (Hashimoto's disease). If pituitary activity is normal thyroid underactivity causes increased TSH secretion, and this may cause thyroid enlargement and goitre formation.

The clinical manifestations of hypothyroidism are those of a general reduction of metabolism. Thus, there is mental retardation, reduced total body oxygen consumption (basal metabolic rate), constipation, bradycardia with low voltage e.c.g. complexes, and in severe cases a tendency to develop hypothermia or even coma (see Chapter 13.) In addition the hair falls out, the voice becomes croaky, and the skin is characteristically dry and thickened with subcutaneous accumulations of mucopolysaccharide (myxoedema). The mental slowing may lead to the development of psychoses, both depressive and of other types ('myxoedema madness').

In children, thyroid hypofunction causes cretinism, with defective growth and impaired mental development (cf. hypopituitarism).

ADRENAL CORTEX

PHYSIOLOGY

The adrenal cortex produces several steroid hormones, and its secretions have a wide variety of actions; on water and electrolyte balance, on carbohydrate and protein metabolism, and on the body's response to 'stress' of various kinds. Inadequate adrenal cortical secretion represents a very real threat to life; and total adrenalectomy without adequate replacement therapy is rapidly fatal.

It is convenient to classify the adrenal steroids into two main types: glucocorticoids, the action of which is predominantly on carbohydrate and protein metabolism, and mineralocorticoids which act predominantly on water and electrolyte balance. There is however considerable overlap between the two groups. The adrenal gland produces also certain sex hormones (mainly androgens), but the importance of these in man is uncertain.

The main glucocorticoid secreted by the human adrenal is cortisol (hydrocortisone), and the main mineralocorticoid is aldosterone. There is also an appreciable secretion of corticosterone, a hormone with predominantly glycocorticoid activity. Cortisol and corticosterone are produced by the inner zones of the cortex; aldosterone by the outer zone (zona glomerulosa).

Glucocorticoids promote the conversion of protein into glucose (gluconeogenesis), inhibit the peripheral utilisation of glucose (perhaps by antagonising the action of insulin—q.v.), and increase hepatic glycogen deposition. In excess, they cause hyperglycaemia. They have also an action on the cardiovascular system, and are necessary for maintenance of the arterial blood pressure and normal glomerular filtration. And they have a most important, but ill-understood, generalized action on the body to increase its resistance to stress of various kinds—infection, trauma, etc.

The mineralocorticicoids influence the rate of sodium and potassium transport across cell membranes. This is particularly important in the kidneys where aldosterone acts predominantly on the distal tubules to cause increased sodium reabsorption and potassium excretion (see Chapter 7).

The rates of secretion of cortisol and corticosterone are modulated by the level of circulating adrenocorticotrophic hormone (ACTH—see section on pituitary); while the rate of secretion of ACTH is itself controlled by the plasma cortisol concentration (acting on the release of CRF from the hypothalamus—see below). As a result of this negative feedback system the concentration of cortisol in the plasma is normally maintained relatively constant (although with a considerable superimposed diurnal variation—normally highest in the morning—due to a variation of ACTH secretion).

In addition, the hypothalamus can directly influence the rate of ACTH secretion. Under conditions of stress, for example, it secretes increased amounts of corticotrophin releasing factor (CRF) into the hypothalamo-hypophyseal portal vessels, thus causing increased ACTH secretion and an adrenal cortical response.

In contrast, aldosterone secretion is little influenced by ACTH, and continues almost unchanged following hypophysectomy. This operation is not therefore accompanied by the dramatic sodium loss and potassium retention which follows adrenalectomy, but rather by a failure to respond to stressful situations (see section on pituitary).

Aldosterone secretion seems mainly to be influenced by the extracellular fluid volume, and by the plasma concentrations of sodium and (especially) potassium. A decrease of extracellular fluid volume stimulates the release of renin from the juxtaglomerular apparatus of the kidney, this enzyme then acts on angiotensinogen in the blood converting it into angiotensin I which is then converted into the octapeptide angiotensin II. In addition to its vasoconstrictor effect (see section on shock) this hormone causes aldosterone release from the adrenal cortex; and thus, by inducing sodium retention, restores the extracellular fluid volume. (There is also evidence that the release of renin from the kidney is affected by the amount of sodium present in the lumen of the ascending limb of Henle's loop where this approaches the juxtaglomerular apparatus.)

A rise in the plasma potassium concentration causes increased aldosterone secretion by a direct action on the adrenal cortex.

The adrenal steroids are synthesised in situ from cholesterol. They are carried in the blood loosely bound to plasma albumin; cortisol is also carried in combination with the α-globulin transcortin. Only the free forms of the hormones are metabolically active and analysis of the total (bound and unbound) steroid in the peripheral blood may therefore give misleading information about the state of adrenal cortical activity. For example, in pregnancy there is increased transcortin production, but no clinical evidence of adrenal hyperactivity, despite increased adrenal steroid concentrations in the blood (a situation similar to that found with TH and TBG—see earlier).

The adrenal hormones all have relatively short half-lives, and they are metabolized in the liver to inactive metabolites. The liver also conjugates both the unchanged hormones and their metabolites with glucuronic acid, thus rendering them water-soluble and in a form which is readily excreted in the urine (as is the case with bilirubin—q.v.).

Biochemical assessment of adrenal function

In recent years it has become possible to investigate adrenal activity biochemically, and thus to define adrenal misfunction with reasonable precision. It is possible, for example, to measure the plasma concentration of cortisol, and also to measure the rates of urinary excretion of various adrenal steroid degradation products.

Adrenal androgens are excreted in the form of 17 oxo (17 keto) steroids. This measurement is however of little diagnostic value because androgens are derived from the gonads as well as from the adrenals. Cortisol is excreted in the urine as a variety of 17 hydroxy-corticocosteroids (17 OHCS); and measurement of the rate of 17

OHCS excretion can give a useful estimate of the rate of adrenal cortisol production. It is possible also to administer a small dose of radioactive cortisol, and then to measure the subsequent ratio of labelled and unlabelled steroid in the blood, and thereby to estimate the rate of adrenal cortisol production.

By combining these tests with the administration of ACTH it is possible to determine whether a defect of adrenal cortical activity is due to adrenal disease *per se,* or to defective ACTH secretion from the pituitary. And the administration of small amounts of a synthetic steroid such as dexamethasone can be used to determine whether adrenal overactivity is autonomous, due to hyperplasia or tumour formation, or the result of excessive ACTH secretion by the anterior pituitary. (Dexamethasone depresses pituitary ACTH secretion—see section on pituitary; and under normal conditions the administration of this hormone therefore markedly depresses the rate of cortisol secretion from the adrenal cortex. In cases of autonomous adrenal overactivity however, it has little or no effect.)

ADRENAL HYPOFUNCTION

General destruction of the adrenal glands, for example by tuberculosis, or carcinomatosis, or (much the most common) idiopathic, perhaps the result of an autoimmune process, causes Addison's disease. The manifestations of this syndrome are due in part to water and electrolyte imbalance; but the majority are due to lack of adrenal glucocorticoid activity which causes generalized weakness and an inability of the kidneys to deal with a sudden, large water load. In addition there is a tendency to hypoglycaemia from reduced gluconeogenesis, and an increased sensitivity to insulin.

The decreased activity of aldosterone on the renal tubules causes severe sodium loss and potassium retention. The resulting depletion of the extracellular fluid compartment causes arterial hypotension and urea retention from impaired renal blood flow (see Chapter 2). When the defect of adrenal cortical function is due, not to adrenal disease *per se,* but to defect ACTH secretion, mineralocorticoid secretion continues largely unimpaired and the clinical manifestations are considerably less dramatic. Under these circumstances the patient usually shows evidence of a lack of other pituitary trophic hormones (see section on pituitary hypofunction).

Reduction in the levels of circulating plasma corticosteroids allows the unrestrained secretion of ACTH from the anterior pituitary. And since there is considerable structural similarity between ACTH and pituitary melanocyte stimulating hormone (see later) this oversecretion results in melanin deposition in various sites, causing the characteristic cutaneous and buccal pigmentation of Addison's disease.

A patient with impaired adrenal cortical function may be relatively well under normal conditions: but if he is exposed to a sudden physical stress such as a surgical operation, his adrenal glands may be incapable of responding to the increased demand, so that he develops adrenal insufficiency. This condition may occur in the early stages of Addison's disease, or when there is a chronic failure of ACTH secretion as in panhypopituitarism (q.v.); but it is particularly common when adrenal cortical function has been suppressed by the long-term iatrogenic administration of glucocorticoids, for example in the treatment of asthma and rheumatoid arthritis. The manifestations of such an episode of acute adrenal insufficiency (Addisonian crisis) are those of prostration and peripheral circulatory failure (see Chapter 2).

Certain individuals have a congenital deficiency of the enzymes which are responsible for cortisol synthesis. The resulting low levels of cortisol in the peripheral blood cause overproduction of ACTH, which in turn causes adrenal hyperplasia and excessive production of the other adrenal hormones, particularly androgens. The result is virilism in girls and precocious sexual development in boys, often accompanied by evidence of glucocorticoid insufficiency (the adrenogenital syndrome).

PITUITARY

PHYSIOLOGY

Embryologically the pituitary arises from two separate sources: the posterior part of the gland arises as a downgrowth from the developing brain; the anterior part as an upgrowth (Rathke's pouch) from the developing foregut. The adult pituitary lies just below the hypothalamus, with which it is intimately related both anatomically and physiologically.

The anterior pituitary is linked to the hypothalamus by the hypothalamo-hypophyseal portal system of blood vessels. These arise in a capillary plexus in the region of the median eminence, and run down the pituitary stalk to break up into capillaries again in the vicinity of the anterior lobe. Chemicals (releasing factors) are liberated from hypothalamic nerve endings, and are then carried along these portal vessels to influence the secretory activity of the anterior pituitary.

The posterior pituitary is connected with the hypothalamus by neurones which arise in the supraoptic and paraventricular nuclei of the hypothalamus, and run down the pituitary stalk to the posterior lobe. It is thought that, in response to an appropriate stimulus, activity in these neurones causes the liberation of ADH and/or oxytocin into the blood vessels of the posterior pituitary (see section on water balance, where the functions of ADH are considered further).

In man, the anterior pituitary produces at least seven hormones which are all polypeptides or glycoproteins. These hormones may be grouped into: growth hormone (GH) which has a generalized action on body metabolism, stimulating growth; melanocyte stimulating hormone (MSH) which influences skin pigmentation, although its precise role in man is uncertain (but see section on Addison's disease); the trophic hormones which control activity in various other endocrine glands—adrenocorticotrophic hormone (corticotrophin, ACTH), thyroid stimulating hormone (TSH), and the hormones which are concerned with the control of sexual function—follicle stimulating hormone (FSH), luteinising hormone (LH) and prolactin.

The rate of secretion (and perhaps of synthesis) of these various hormones is controlled by the activity of the appropriate releasing factor (or, in the case of prolactin and MSH, inhibiting factor): growth hormone releasing factor (GHRF), thyroid stimulating hormone releasing factor (TSHRF), corticotrophin releasing factor (CRF), luteinising hormone releasing factor (LHRF), follicle stimulating hormone releasing factor (FSHRF), prolactin inhibiting factor (PIF), and melanocyte stimulating hormone inhibiting factor (MIF). These factors are all low molecular weight polypeptides: TSHRF, for example, is a tripeptide.

The factors which affect the rate of GH release are incompletely understood. It is known to be secreted in response to exercise and to stress of various kinds, and also in response to fasting, to reductions in blood glucose concentration, and amino acid infusions.

The rate of release of the various trophic hormones is controlled by negative feedback mechanisms, by which the release of the trophic hormone is dependent on the concentration in the peripheral blood of the controlled hormone (i.e. the hormone whose rate of secretion is controlled by the trophic hormone). Thus, an increase in the level of cortisol in the peripheral blood causes a decrease in the rate of secretion of ACTH; and a decrease in cortisol concentration causes increased ACTH secretion. Similar mechanisms exist with the other trophic hormones.

In the case of TSH it appears that the feedback is mediated directly by the action of thyroid hormone on the anterior pituitary; in the case of ACTH and the gonad-controlling hormones, the feedback is predominantly to the hypothalamus. In addition, there may be short feedback loops by which hypothalamic hormone release has a direct effect on the rate of secretion of hypothalamic releasing factors.

The hypothalamus, via its releasing factors, may affect pituitary hormone secretion so as to override the feedback systems considered above. This is seen in the case of ACTH, where physical stress causes increased pituitary secretion (see section on adrenal gland); and in the case of the sex hormones, where the cyclic waxing and waning of FSH and LH release which characterises the female reproductive cycle is the result of rhythmic variations in hypothalamic activity. (In contrast, the rate of secretion of these hormones in the male is relatively constant.)

GH stimulates the transport of amino acids into cells and their subsequent synthesis into protein. At the same time it inhibits fat synthesis, and causes the release of fatty acids from adipose tissue. The uptake of glucose into cells is also inhibited, with a consequent decreased sensitivity to the blood sugar-lowering effect of insulin. In the whole animal, of course, the most obvious action of GH is to stimulate growth: excessive secretion before epiphyseal closure results in giantism, after epiphyseal fusion in acromegaly. The latter condition is commonly accompanied by diabetes mellitus (q.v.). The growth rate of pituitary dwarfs can be increased to normal, or even above, by the administration of GH.

The effects of prolactin are complex. In addition to its obvious action in promoting lactation it appears to have a variety of other actions, including those on the kidneys where it causes water and electrolyte retention, both directly and by potentiating the actions of aldosterone and ADH.

Assessment of pituitary function

Deficient pituitary function is normally reflected in biochemical evidence of hyposecretion from its various target organs (see earlier). Evidence of pituitary hypofunction may also be obtained by the administration of the drug metyrapone. This interferes with the adrenal synthesis of cortisol at the stage where desoxycortisol is converted to cortisol; and the resulting decrease in the level of circulating cortisol normally stimulates the pituitary to secrete increased amounts of ACTH which then cause the adrenal cortex to produce large amounts of steroid—not of cortisol however because the necessary enzymes are inactive, but of cortisol precursors whose metabolic products appear in the urine as 17 OHCS (see earlier). When there is pituitary underactivity the gland is unable to increase its ACTH production in response to the reduction of plasma cortisol concentration; and the administration of metyrapone is not then accompanied by an increase of urinary 17 OHCS.

HYPOPITUITARISM

It is difficult to present a concise account of the clinical manifestations of anterior pituitary underactivity. The pituitary gland has a wide range of metabolic activities which are carried out in a very small region of the body; and a destructive lesion of this gland may be accompanied either by generalized hypopituitarism, or by a deficiency in the function of one cell type only, or by overactivity of unaffected cells resulting in e.g. increased ACTH secretion and Cushing's syndrome.

Generalized destruction of the pituitary gives rise to the signs and symptoms of panhypopituitarism. In the past this was commonly due to infarction of the gland after a period of postpartum shock (Sheehan's syndrome) but this is now rarely seen, It may arise also as a result of trauma, infection, or a chromophobe cell adenoma, or other local tumour. Space-occupying lesions of the pituitary are commonly associated with manifestations of raised intracranial pressure, and by visual defects from pressure on the region of the optic chiasma.

In adult hypopituitarism (Simmonds' disease) there are signs of a lack of the various pituitary trophic hormones, with hypothyroidism, hypogonadism, and adrenal insufficiency (but not with the marked electrolyte disturbances which characterize Addison's disease—q.v.). There is marked cutaneous pallor, perhaps due to deficient MSH secretion (cf. the marked pigmentation of adrenal insufficiency). In Sheehan's syndrome a difficult confinement is followed by failure of lactation and persistent amenorrhoea, with gradual appearance of the other stigmata of hypopituitarism.

In children, pituitary hyposecretion causes dwarfism and pituitary infantilism, in which there is a failure of growth and of sexual development, although (in contrast to what is found in thyroid underactivity—q.v.) mental development is relatively normal. In Fröhlich's syndrome (dystrophia adiposogenitalis) infantilism is associated with obesity, and sometimes with temperature and/or sleep disturbances as a result of associated hypothalamic dysfunction.

Patients with inadequately treated hypopituitarism are particularly likely to go into coma following some relatively minor stress; but the relative etiological roles played by hypoglycaemia (due to increased insulin sensitivity), hypothermia (due to hypothyroidism), and fluid and electrolyte disturbances (due to adrenal insufficiency) are uncertain. In adults, GH despite its widespread metabolic effects, appears to be relatively inessential, because patients with hypopituitarism can be kept in good health by replacement therapy with adrenal corticosteroids, thyroid hormone, and the appropriate sex hormones.

INSULIN

PHYSIOLOGY

Insulin is a small molecular weight protein (mol. wt. $\simeq$ 6000) produced by the β-cells of the pancreatic islets. The amino acid composition of insulins from different species varies slightly. Fortunately, however, these differences are slight; and insulin is therefore only weakly antigenic, and bovine and porcine insulins may be used clinically in man.

The chief factor which determines the rate of insulin release from the pancreas is the blood glucose concentration. The membranes of the islet cells are freely permeable to glucose, and a rise in blood glucose concentration causes increased insulin secretion from these cells; a fall causes decreased secretion.

There are in addition several ancillary factors which affect pancreatic insulin release, but the relative importance of these factors is uncertain. Orally administered glucose is particularly effective in stimulating insulin release, suggesting that a gastrointestinal hormone may be involved—secretin, pancreozymin and intestinal glucagon have all been suggested for this role. Insulin secretion may also be stimulated by ketone bodies, by sympathetic stimulation and by the sulphonylureas tolbutamide and chlorpropamide, which are used clinically especially in the treatment of mature-onset diabetes (see later).

The actions of insulin are many: the chief one however seems to be its blood sugar-lowering effect, which is mediated by its action on cell membranes, enhancing the cellular uptake of glucose, and stimulating peripheral glucose utilisation, particularly in fat and muscle. In addition, there is depression of the hepatic breakdown of glycogen and of hepatic gluconeogenesis, and stimulation of protein, glycogen and triglyceride synthesis in various parts of the body. The net result of these various actions is a decrease in the circulating levels of glucose and free fatty acid in the peripheral blood.

The pancreatic islets also produce glucagon. This is a polypeptide with actions which are generally antagonistic to those of insulin, causing increased hepatic glycogenolysis and hyperglycaemia. A similar substance (intestinal glucagon) is produced by the duodenal mucosa.

The glucose tolerance test

The body's ability to deal with a carbohydrate load may conveniently be assessed by performing a glucose tolerance test, i.e. by measuring the blood glucose concentration at intervals after a glucose load, usually 50g given orally. In a normal person the blood glucose concentration during the test should not exceed about 8 mmol/l (150 mg/100 ml), and should have returned to its fasting level within two hours; and, provided the renal threshold is normal, no glucose should spill over into the urine.

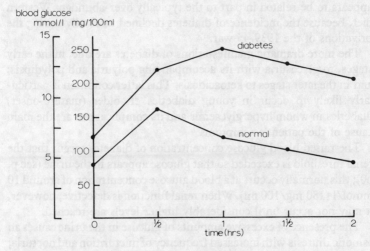

Fig 18. Normal and diabetic glucose tolerance curves.

In a patient with fully developed diabetes the fasting blood glucose is above normal (about 4.5 mmol/l; 80 mg/100 ml), the peak level is considerably above 8 mmol/l and usually exceeds the renal threshold, and the return to the fasting value is greatly delayed (Fig. 18). In patients with mild diabetes the resting and peak values may not be greatly elevated, but the time course of the response is prolonged.

DIABETES MELLITUS

The syndrome of hyperglycaemia, glycosuria, and ketoacidosis (diabetes mellitus, cf. diabetes insipidus which is due to defective activity of ADH—see section on water balance) arises whenever there is an absolute or relative insulin deficiency. Thus, diabetes may arise when there is deficient pancreatic insulin secretion, as after pancreatectomy, in pancreatitis and haemochromatosis (q.v.), idiopathically, or when there is a loss of peripheral sensitivity to insulin, due perhaps to the action of a circulating insulin antagonist. Alternatively, diabetes may occur when there is excessive secretion of one of the hormones which antagonize the peripheral actions of insulin, e.g. of GH in acromegaly,

of corticosteroids in Cushing's syndrome or iatrogenically administered, or of catecholamines from a phaeochromocytoma.

It has been estimated that around one million persons in Great
Britain suffer from diabetes mellitus, although in about half the
disease is still subclinical, i.e., may be detected by 'screening' tests but
does not give rise to significant clinical symptoms. This high incidence
appears to be related in part to the typically over-abundant Western
diet, because the incidence of diabetes declined markedly during the
privations of the 1939-45 war.

The more dramatic manifestations of diabetes are due, in the early
stages, to glycosuria with its accompanying polyuria and polydipsia;
and in the later stages to ketoacidosis. This latter condition is particularly likely to occur in young diabetics cf. older (mature-onset)
diabetics in whom hyperglycaemia and its complications are the main
cause of the patient's symptoms.

The raised blood glucose concentration of diabetes means that the
renal threshold is exceeded so that glucose appears in the urine (see p.
p0); this normally occurs at a blood glucose concentration of around 10
mmol/l (180 mg/100 ml). When renal function is defective, however,
it may not occur until considerably higher levels are reached.

The presence of excessive amounts of glucose in the urine causes an
osmotic diuresis with increased frequency of micturition and nocturia;
and the accompanying loss of water and electrolytes causes thirst and
polydipsia, and in severe cases extracellular fluid depletion (see section
on sodium depletion) which may be sufficiently severe to produce
circulatory collapse (see section on peripheral circulatory failure).

The other important consequence of defective peripheral carbohydrate utilization is ketoacidósis. The body normally metabolizes fatty
acids by progressively splitting them into 2C fragments (acetyl
coenzyme A, acetyl CoA) which then combine with oxaloacetic acid to
enter the Krebs tricarboxylic acid cycle, in which they are converted to
carbon dioxide and water, with the release of energy in the form of
ATP. The chief source of oxaloacetic acid is normally pyruvic acid
derived from carbohydrate metabolism ('fats are burned in a carbohydrate furnace'). The absence of effective carbohydrate metabolism (as
in diabetes) therefore impairs fatty acid metabolism also, and the
acetyl CoA molecules then combine to form ketone bodies—acetone,
acetoacetic acid, and β-hydroxybutyric acid which build up in the
blood to cause a severe metabolic derangement—ketoacidosis. (A
similar, but less dramatic, abnormality of fat metabolism may occur
during starvation where there is also reduced carbohydrate utilization.)

The manifestations of ketoacidosis are protean including: weakness, nausea, vomiting, abdominal pain (especially in children), and ultimately impairment of consciousness (diabetic coma). Ketone bodies are excreted in the breath, giving it a characteristic odour of acetone, and in the urine where they may be detected by the appropriate tests. Their presence in the blood also causes osmotic transfer of water from the intracellular fluid compartment, with resulting intracellular dehydration; and their excretion in the urine exacerbates the osmotic diuresis and resulting dehydration caused by the glycosuria. There is a metabolic acidosis with compensatory respiratory alkalosis (see section on acid-base balance).

In the adult type of diabetes there is less tendency to the development of ketoacidosis; but the osmotic diuresis caused by the glycosuria may cause considerable dehydration and hypernatraemia with impairment of consciousness (hyperosmolar diabetic coma).

There are also other, less specific manifestations of diabetes. Defective protein and fat synthesis causes loss of weight and muscular wasting; the presence of sugar in the urine encourages genitourinary infection, particularly candidiasis ('thrush'); and there are a number of relatively frequent complications, for example: angiopathy, nephropathy, retinopathy and neuropathy. The high incidence of these complications is presumably related to the abnormal fat and carbohydrate metabolism because there is evidence that their incidence may be reduced by careful long-term maintenance of the patient's blood glucose concentration near to normal values.

FURTHER READING

Alexander L 1977 Pituitary problems. Practitioner 218: 532
Anon 1970 Cyclic AMP: the second messenger. Lancet ii: 1119
Anon 1976 Ectopic secretion by tumours. Lancet i: 1300
Catt K J 1971 An ABC of endocrinology. The Lancet Ltd, London
Cudworth A G 1976 The aetiology of diabetes mellitus. British Journal of Hospital Medicine 16: 207
Dains J C, Hipkin L J 1977 Clinical endocrine pathology. Blackwell, Oxford
Davies A G 1972 Thyroid physiology. British Medical Journal i: 206
Evered D, Hall R 1972 Hypothyroidism. British Medical Journal i: 290
Fraser R 1972 Metabolic disorders in diabetes. British Medical Journal iv: 591
Hall R, Anderson J, Smart G A, Besser M 1974 Fundamentals of clinical endocrinology, 2nd edn. Pitman Medical, London
Hartog M 1972 Hypoadrenalism. British Medical Journal i: 679
Harvard C W H 1973 The investigation of adrenal function. In: Frontiers of medicine. Heinemann, London
Harvard C W H 1974 Which test of thyroid function? British Medical Journal i: 553
Harvard C W H 1975 The assessment of thyroid function. British Journal of Hospital Medicine 14: 239
Irvine W J, Toft A D 1977 Diagnosing adrenal insufficiency. Practitioner 218: 539

Jenkins J S 1972 The hypothalamus. British Medical Journal ii: 99
Nabarro J D N 1972 Pituitary tumours and hypopituitarism. British Medical
    Journal i: 492
Ryan W G 1976 Endocrine disorders: a pathophysiological approach. Lloyd-Luke,
    London
Singer B 1972 Adrenal corticosteroids-physiological considerations. British Medical
    Journal i: 36

11

Osteoporosis and osteomalacia

The body of a 70 kg man contains about 1100g of calcium, of which the vast majority (more than 99 per cent) is contained within the bony skeleton. However, despite the small absolute amount of calcium carried in the plasma, several important physiological processess, e.g. bone formation, blood coagulation (q.v.), neuromuscular transmission, and cardiac contraction depend fundamentally on the plasma concentration of (ionized) calcium. This concentration is normally maintained within narrow limits (2.2 to 2.8 mmol/l; 9 to 11 mg/100 ml) by the activity of two hormones, parathyroid hormone and calcitonin. In general, these have opposing actions: parathyroid hormone promotes calcium removal from the bones and thus raises the plasma calcium concentration; calcitonin has the opposite effect.

This chapter is concerned chiefly with the role of calcium in bone formation, and with the skeletal defects known as osteomalacia and osteoporosis. Although a somewhat dogmatic approach is adopted, and the two condititons are treated as completely separate entities, it should be stressed that the details of their pathogenesis are only partially understood, and there is evidence that calcium deficiency may be a causative factor in both.

PHYSIOLOGY

The normal concentrations of calcium and phosphate in the plasma are, respectively, about 2.5 mmol/l (10 mg/100 ml) and 1.6 mmol/l (5 mg/100 ml). The calcium is in two main forms: part (about 40 per cent) is carried in combination with plasma albumin, the remainder is carried in solution as the free, ionized form. It is this latter component which is responsible for its various metabolic activities; but it is the total calcium which is measured by generally available biochemical techniques.

On a normal diet, the body's calcium intake is in the region of 1000mg/day, chiefly in the form of milk and milk products. Of this intake, about 100mg/day (range 50 to 400 mg) is actively absorbed from the jejunum and duodenum under the influence of vitamin D (see below), and then either retained in the body or excreted in the urine, depending on whether or not the body is in calcium balance. The remainder of the ingested calcium (about 900 mg) is excreted in the faeces. (Calcium also enters the gut with the digestive secretions. On a normal diet, however, the net effect on calcium balance of this additional load is nil—Fig. 19.)

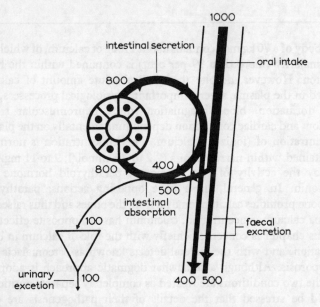

Fig 19 Quantitative aspects of calcium balance (after Jackson, 1962). (Figures in mg/24 h.)

When the body is in calcium balance, urinary loss is equal to the net rate of calcium absorption from the gut. When the body is in negative balance, urinary calcium excretion exceeds net intestinal absorption, and vice versa when the patient is in positive balance, as during a period of rapid growth.

Vitamin D
The absorption of calcium from the gut depends on the activity of vitamin D. In the absence of this vitamin, very little calcium absorption occurs, however high the calcium intake; conversely, in the presence of adequate amounts of vitamin D, it is virtually impossible to cause calcium deficiency by dietary means alone.

The naturally-occurring form of vitamin D is cholecalciferol (vitamin D_3). The form which is used therapeutically is vitamin D_2 (calciferol). Vitamin D occurs particularly in fish-liver oils and in dairy produce—milk, eggs, butter, etc. It is also formed in the skin by the action of sunlight on 7-dehydrocholesterol. This production is important, because even on a normal diet, vitamin D deficiency can occur in dark-skinned races living in sunlight-deficient northern cities. In Britain vitamin D is artificially added to margarine.

The chief action of vitamin D is to promote the absorption of calcium from the upper part of the small intestine. It probably has also a slight effect on the renal tubules, causing a small increase in urinary phosphate excretion. In a patient with calcium-deficient bones, vitamin D promotes calcium deposition and skeletal recalcification; but, in a normal person, the administration of excessive amounts of this vitamin may cause skeletal demineralization, with hypercalciuria and metastatic deposition of calcium in soft tissues.

Recently it has become clear that vitamin D metabolism is considerably more complex than was formerly thought. Cholecalciferol is first converted in the liver into 25-hydroxycholecalciferol; and then, in the kidney, this substance is further hydroxylated to 1,25 dihydroxycholecalciferol. This is the active metabolite. The rate of renal conversion of 25-hydroxycholecalciferol into 1,25 dihydroxycholecalciferol is under the control of a variety of factors, particularly the level of parathyroid hormone in the peripheral blood. Thus, a decrease in the level of circulating calcium causes release of parathyroid hormone (see later), this enhances the renal production of 1,25 dihydroxycholecalciferol, and thereby causes an increase in the absorption of calcium from the gut, so restoring the plasma calcium level.

Clinically, vitamin D deficiency gives rise to rickets in children, and to osteomalacia in adults (see later).

Control of plasma calcium concentration
The concentration of calcium in the plasma is finely controlled by two hormones—parathyroid hormone and calcitonin.

Parathyroid hormone
Parathyroid hormone is a polypeptide which, in the presence of vitamin D, promotes calcium resorption from the bones, and therefore results in an increase of plasma calcium concentration. It also influences the rate of production of 1,25 dihydroxycholecalciferol (see above). The normal stimulus for the release of parathyroid hormone is a fall of plasma (ionized) calcium concentration; the resulting hormonal secretion initiates a negative feedback process, and restores the plasma calcium concentration towards normal. No parathyroid hor-

mone is secreted when the plasma calcium concentration exceeds about 3 mmol/1 (12 mg/100 ml).

Parathyroid hormone also increases renal phosphate excretion by decreasing the tubular reabsorption of this ion; and at the same time it increases renal calcium reabsorption, although, because of increased plasma calcium levels, renal calcium excretion is usually increased rather than decreased. Parathyroid hormone may also enhance calcium absorption from the small intestine.

Excessive secretion of parathyroid hormone (hyperparathyroidism) is thus manifested by hypercalcaemia and hypophosphataemia, accompanied by increased urinary excretion of both calcium and phosphate ions, and by a negative calcium balance. In addition, there is extensive skeletal demineralization and extraosseous calcium deposition.

Calcitonin
Calcitonin is also a polypeptide, produced in the thyroid gland ('thyrocalcitonin'). It is secreted in response to a rise of plasma calcium concentration, and its release is inhibited by a lowered plasma calcium level. The action of calcitonin opposes that of parathyroid hormone; it lowers the plasma calcium concentration by inhibiting bone calcium resorption and (to a lesser extent) by inhibiting tubular calcium reabsorption.

Contrary to what might be expected, calcitonin seems to be of little clinical use in the treatment of osteoporosis; but it does appear to be of value in Paget's disease.

Bone formation
Bone consists of an uncalcified matrix supporting an orderly array of minute crystals of various calcium salts (chiefly in the form of calcium phosphate known as hydroxyapatite), thereby forming a very rigid, very light structure. The calcium in the bones is not inert, but is in dynamic equilibrium with the ionized calcium of the blood; bone is continually being laid down and resorbed, processes which are associated respectively with the activity of two types of cell—osteoblasts and osteoclasts.

The first step in new bone formation is the laying down of the collagenous matrix, osteoid which is secreted by the osteoblasts. This matrix then becomes calcified by the deposition of calcium phosphate, a process which requires that the local solubility product of calcium and phosphate $[Ca^{2+}] \times [PO'''_4]$ is exceeded, so that calcium phosphate can precipitate out of solution. It has been postulated that osteoblasts secrete alkaline phosphatase, which hydrolyses phosphate esters in the vicinity of the collagenous matrix, and thus raises the calcium/phosphate solubility product above the critical level at which precipitation occurs. However, the whole process of bone formation is ill-understood, and is likely to remain so until techniques become available for measuring the pH at the site of new bone formation. (The critical solubility product above which precipitation of calcium phosphate occurs is of course a function of the local hydrogen ion concentration.)

OSTEOMALACIA

Osteomalacia (softening of the bones) arises as a result of a reduction of the skeletal mineral content, with no accompanying reduction of organic matrix. The condition thus contrasts with osteoporosis (atrophy of the bones—see later) in which there is a reduction of both skeletal components, organic and inorganic. In children the bones are still growing, and conditions which in adults would cause osteomalacia give rise to rickets, with rather different clinical manifestations.

The bony abnormalities of osteomalacia are accompanied by an increased plasma concentration of alkaline phosphatase, the enzyme concerned in osteoblastic activity. (This enzyme is excreted by the liver, therefore its plasma concentration is raised also when there is defective hepatic function, especially obstructive jaundice—q.v.) In osteomalacia from vitamin D deficiency (see below) there is a reduction of the plasma concentrations of both calcium and phosphate (the latter from parathyroid overactivity), and a low urinary calcium excretion. Osteomalacia from hyperparathyroidism (see below) is, however, accompanied by a marked increase of plasma calcium concentration.

PATHOGENESIS

Vitamin D deficiency

Vitamin D deficiency causes defective calcium absorption, and results in a reduced calcium concentration in the plasma, and defective skeletal mineralization. Osteomalacia due purely to dietary deficiency of vitamin D is, however, rare in this country*, and patients with skeletal abnormalities which are apparently due to this cause usually have an added element of intestinal malabsorption (q.v.). An exception is the rapidly growing child, whose requirements of vitamin D are relatively great; under these circumstances rickets is by no means unknown, particularly in undernourished immigrant children in northern cities (see above).

*It does, however, appear to be becoming more common—a sad commentary on the Nation's health services.

Osteomalacia from vitamin D deficiency, whether dietary or secondary to intestinal malabsorption, is readily treated by small doses of vitamin D (given parenterally in the malabsorption case), and is therefore often known as vitamin D sensitive osteomalacia, in contrast to the vitamin D resistant form (see below).

Renal disease

Osteomalacia may accompany two types of renal disease; renal tubular acidosis and other congenital tubular defects (rare) and chronic azotaemic renal failure (q.v.) In both cases the condition is very resistant to treatment with vitamin D, although massive doses may be effective.

In renal tubular dysfunction there is excessive loss of phosphate in the urine, commonly accompanied by abnormal renal handling of amino acids, glucose and hydrogen ions. Biochemically, the patient has a metabolic acidosis and hypophosphataemia, but a relatively normal plasma calcium level.

In chronic renal failure, renal phosphate clearance may be severely reduced, with consequent hyperphosphataemia, hypocalcaemia, and impaired skeletal mineral deposition, due partly to excessive parathyroid activity. This condition is very resistant to treatment, although it may be reversed by very large doses of vitamin D (see section on renal failure).

Hyperparathyroidism

Osteomalacia may occur as part of the syndrome of hyperparathyroidism. Oversecretion of parathyroid hormone occurs in response to abnormalities of the plasma calcium concentration; it may be due also to autonomous oversecretion, as a result of either simple hyperplasia or tumour formation (usually adenomatous). Occasionally, a patient who has had years of parathyroid overactivity, due for example, to the malabsorption syndrome (q.v.) develops autonomous ('tertiary') hyperparathyroidism. The difference between secondary oversecretion and autonomous overactivity is, of course, that the latter condition cannot be reversed by raising the plasma calcium concentration.

Hyperparathyroidism causes hypercalcaemia, increased loss of calcium and phosphate in the urine and characteristic bony abnormalities (osteitis fibrosa). The hypercalciuria may cause renal stone formation; while the increased plasma calcium concentration may result in calcium deposition around the renal tubules (nephrocalcinosis), and in soft tissues generally.

CLINICAL MANIFESTATIONS OF OSTEOMALACIA

Osteomalacia affects the whole skeleton, whereas osteoporosis (q.v.) tends to affect only the bones of the axial skeleton (spine and limb girdles). In osteomalacia the bones are painful, tender and soft, and may bend under the influence of gravity. On X-ray examination, they commonly show areas of rarefaction ('pseudofractures') running transversely across part of their thickness. These areas of rarefaction are known as Milkman's or Looser's zones, and are seen particularly at the upper end of the humerus and femur and at the lower end of the tibia. In addition, the patient may have low back pain from spinal abnormalities.

In childhood osteomalacia (rickets) the growing ends of the bones, particularly of the radius and the costochondral junctions become swollen due to the abnormal formation of uncalcified osteoid. These swellings give rise to the typical 'rickety rosary' and to bossing of the skull. The softened bones of the rachitic child are particularly liable to bend, causing bowing of the legs or knock-knee, and pelvic deformities which may give rise to difficulties in future child-bearing.

In osteomalacia from hyperparathyroidism the plasma calcium concentration may be raised considerably above the normal range to as high as 5 mmol/l (20 mg/100 ml). And, in addition to metastatic calcification in the kidneys and elsewhere, such hypercalcaemia may give rise to symptoms such as anorexia, vomiting, mental apathy, muscular hypotonia, and peptic ulceration. There is also usually marked polyuria, due partly to osmotic diuresis and partly to the fact that the renal tubules are (for some unknown reason) unresponsive to the action of antidiuretic hormone. The skeleton may show specific (and diagnostic) X-ray appearances, with subperiosteal erosions, multiple bone cysts and the characteristic 'pepperpot skull'.

OSTEOPOROSIS

In osteoporosis the composition of the skeleton is normal, but a reduced amount of bony tissue is present; the defect is quantitative rather than qualitative. Osteoporosis also contrasts with osteomalacia in that the plasma levels of calcium, phosphorus, and alkaline phosphatase are normal.

PATHOGENESIS

In most cases the precise biochemical cause of osteoporosis is unknown, although there are some clinical conditions which are commonly associated with this abnormality.

Disuse might be expected to result in a reduction in the amount of skeletal material present in the body; and it is well recognized that osteoporosis may occur as a result of prolonged bed rest, particularly in elderly patients.* Osteoporosis occurs in old age, even without prolonged bed rest; this is particularly so in postmenopausal women (postmenopausal osteoporosis) and in very old men (senile osteoporosis). It occurs also in conditions in which there is abnormal protein metabolism, for example in the malabsorption syndrome (q.v.) and in Cushing's syndrome and hypercortism from excessive iatrogenic steroid administration. Osteoporosis may be seen also in thyrotoxicosis.

CLINICAL MANIFESTATIONS OF OSTEOPOROSIS

Quite severe, radiologically-confirmed osteoporosis may be present in the almost complete absence of clinical manifestations. The atrophied bones of these patients are, however, particularly prone to fracture, even with minor trauma; this is particularly the case with the vertebral bodies and the femoral necks. These fractures heal readily. The intermittent pain of such bony injuries contrasts markedly with the persistent, nagging pain of osteomalacia and some other forms of bone disease, e.g. secondary neoplasia. Vertebral involvement may give rise to low back pain and a progressive decrease of stature.

The decreased bone density of osteoporosis is readily seen radiologically, with changes in the trabecular pattern of the bones and cortical thinning. In the vertebral column there may be widening of the intervertebral spaces and wedging of the vertebral bodies from spontaneous fractures.

*And also in astronauts, as a result of the absence of the effects of gravity.

FURTHER READING

Anon 1970 Osteoporosis. Lancet i: 180
Anon 1973 The need for vitamin-D supplements. Lancet i: 1105
Anon 1978 'One-alpha'. Lancet i: 973
Campbell E J M, Dickinson C J, Slater J D H 1974 Clinical Physiology, 4th edn. Blackwell, Oxford, ch 9
Catt K J 1970 Hormonal control of calcium homeostasis. Lancet ii: 255
Conacher W D H 1973 Metabolic bone disease in the elderly. Practitioner 210: 351
Evans I M A 1979 Calcitonin treatment of Paget's disease. Lancet ii: 1232
Hoffman W S 1970 The biochemistry of clinical medicine, 4th edn. Year Book Medical Publishers, Chicago, ch 12
Hosking D J 1977 Diseases of the urinary system: renal osteodystrophy. British Medical Journal ii: 110
Irving J T 1973 Calcium and phosphorous metabolism. Academic Press, New York and London

Jackson W P U 1962 Calcium balance made easy. Lancet i: 849

Kodicek E 1974 The story of vitamin D, from vitamin to hormone. Lancet i: 325

Nordin B E C 1973 Metabolic bone and stone disease. Churchill Livingstone, Edinburgh and London

Rasmussen H, Bordier P 1974 The physiological and cellular basis of metabolic bone disease. Williams and Wilkins, Baltimore

Reeve J 1979 Therapeutic applications of vitamin D analogues. British Medical Journal 2: 888

Smith R 1979 Biochemical disorders of the skeleton. Butterworths, London

Tomlinson S 1978 The parathyroids. British Journal of Hospital Medicine 19: 40

Watson L 1973 Endocrine bone disease. Practitioner 210: 376

Eills M R 1971 Disorders of calcium homeostasis. British Journal of Hospital Medicine 6: 65

Wills M R 1973 Calcium homeostasis in health and disease. In: Baron D N, Compston N, Dawson A M (ed) Recent advances in medicine, 16th edn. Churchill Livingstone, Edinburgh and London

12

Disorders of fluid and electrolyte balance

Disorders of fluid and electrolyte balance may complicate a variety of disease processes. The consequences of such disorders depend not only on the magnitude of the deficit or excess, but on its nature—on whether it involves solely the intravascular compartment, the intravascular compartment plus the interstitial fluid, or the entire body water, intracellular as well as extracellular.

Some 70 per cent of the normal adult male body is composed of water, distributed somewhat as follows:

	litres
Intracellular fluid	35
Extracellular fluid	
interstitial fluid	12
plasma	3
	——
	50

The percentage is somewhat less in the female, due chiefly to the greater proportion of body weight composed of fat, which is relatively water-free; it is somewhat greater in the infant.

The composition of the intra and extracellular fluids differs considerably (Fig. 20). These differences are important in maintaining cellular function and are produced by the activity of a sodium/potassium 'pump' which actively transports these ions across cell membranes. The ionic compositions of the two components of the extracellular fluid are similar, except that plasma contains about 70 g/l of protein which, by the Donnan effect, causes small (and unimportant) ionic differences across the vascular membrane.

In each compartment the sum of the anions and the sum of the cations must balance so as to maintain electrical neutrality. The chief intracellular cation is potassium, balanced mainly by protein and phosphate anions; the chief extracellular cation is sodium, balanced by chloride, bicarbonate and (in the blood) protein (Fig. 20).

Potassium loss affects mainly the intracellular fluid (i.c.f.); it is consequently difficult to diagnose, because serious abnormalities of intracellular composition may be reflected hardly at all in the composition of the extracellular fluid (which is normally all that is available for biochemical analysis). Because sodium is the main extracellular cation, a sodium deficit reduces the volume of the entire extracellular fluid (e.c.f.)—interstitial fluid and plasma. Such a reduction of e.c.f. volume has, however, less serious consequences than the loss of an equivalent amount of fluid from the intravascular compartment alone (see section on haemorrhage). In the same way, the consequences of a pure water deficit are less serious than those of a similar loss of e.c.f., because pure water loss is spread throughout the whole body water (50 l), rather than being limited to the 15 or so litres of e.c.f.

WATER

PHYSIOLOGY

Water intake
In lower species, water intake is regulated solely by the thirst mechanism, and by water availability. An increase of crystalloid osmotic pressure in the body fluids gives rise to the sensation of thirst, thus inducing increased water intake, and so restoring body water content to normal. (In addition, ADH secretion is increased, so minimizing renal water loss—see later.)

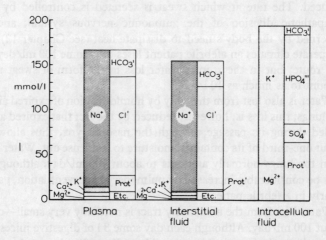

Fig. 20 Electrolyte composition of plasma, interstitial fluid and intracellular fluid (after Gamble, 1954).

This primitive mechanism is present also in man, but is overlaid by a variety of psychological and social factors, so that fluid intake usually exceeds that required merely to prevent thirst. This excess water intake must be excreted by the kidneys.

The precise physiological mechanism(s) which underlie the sensation of thirst are unknown. In lower animals, and probably in man, there are hypothalamic receptors which respond to changes in the tonicity of their environment. The sensation may be related also to changes in the volume or composition of the saliva. Hypovolaemia, such as accompanies acute haemorrhage (q.v.) also produces thirst; the location of the volume receptors which initiate this mechanism is not known with certainty, but may be the left atrium.

Water loss

Water loss occurs in the urine, and from the skin, the lungs, and, to a small extent, the gastrointestinal tract.

Cutaneous water loss is partly by diffusion through the outer layers of the skin (insensible water loss) and partly in the form of sweat. The former is inevitable, and its extent is determined by the skin temperature and the humidity of the environment. In temperate climates water loss by this route amounts to 300 to 500 ml/day.

Sweat is a dilute aqueous solution of sodium chloride in a concentration roughly equal to one-half that in the plasma. Sweating therefore involves loss of sodium as well as water, although in a heat-acclimatized subject the sodium content of the sweat may be somewhat reduced. The rate at which sweat is secreted is controlled by the sympathetic division of the autonomic nervous system, and is governed by the body's need to dissipate heat (see Chapter 13). In temperate climates an afebrile patient loses only some 100 ml/day by this route; but in the tropics water loss in the form of sweat may amount to as much as 10 l/day.

Water is also lost from the body by humidification of expired air in the lungs; this loss is, however, reduced by the fact that expired air is cooled during its passage through the nasopharynx, thus allowing about one-third of its contained moisture to condense out. Water loss from the lungs normally amounts to about 700 ml/day, although it may be considerably increased by pulmonary hyperventilation, particularly in a febrile patient.

Water loss from the alimentary tract is normally very small—only about 100 ml/day. Although each day some 8 l of digestive juices are secreted into the intestinal lumen, all but 100 to 200 ml are reabsorbed before the start of the pelvic colon. Intestinal fluid reabsorption is an active process over which the body has little or no control; and excessive water intake may, in the presence of defective renal function, lead to signs and symptoms of 'water intoxication' (see later). Gastrointestinal water loss is considerably increased in diarrhoea, and particularly in cholera.

Renal water loss is partly under hormonal control and partly inevitable ('obligatory'). On a normal diet, the kidneys have to excrete daily about 1000 mOs of ingested solutes and metabolic waste products. The maximum urinary concentration is normally about 1300 mOs/l, therefore the excretion of this water load necessitates a renal water loss of about 700 ml/day. In the presence of defective renal function, however, when the renal concentrating ability is reduced, the obligatory urine volume may be considerably increased (see Fig. 21).

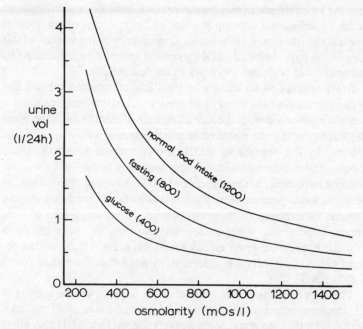

Fig. 21. Urine flow required to excrete different solute loads at different urine osmolarities. (Figures in mOs.)

Fasting reduces the osmotic load on the renal excretory mechanism, and therefore the obligatory urine volume, but excretion of the products of protein breakdown still requires a urine flow of about 0.6 l/day. The administration of glucose to a fasting subject minimizes protein breakdown, reducing the osmotic load to be excreted to about 400 mOs/day. With normal renal concentrating power this requires an obligatory water loss of some 300 ml/day (see Fig. 21), but considerably more when renal concentrating ability is impaired by disease (see section on renal failure).

The amount of water excreted by the kidney each minute in excess of that needed to eliminate the body's excretory solute load as urine which is isotonic with the plasma is known as the 'free water clearance'. This parameter is controlled by the plasma ADH (antidiuretic hormone) concentration so as to maintain e.c.f. osmolarity within the normal range ($\simeq$ 300 mOs/l). (When the urine is hypertonic with respect to the plasma, the calculated free water clearance is negative.)

ADH is produced in the supraoptic and paraventricular nuclei of the hypothalamus, and transported as neurosecretory granules along the pituitary stalk to the posterior lobe of the pituitary. It is discharged into the bloodstream in response to nervous impulses which originate in the hypothalamic supraoptic nucleus. The stimulus which initiates this mechanism is an increase of e.c.f. osmolarity in the vicinity of this area of the hypothalamus. ADH secretion may also be influenced by the activity of 'volume' receptors in the left atrium.

ADH appears to act mainly on the distal convoluted tubules and collecting ducts of the kidney (see section on renal failure). Sodium is actively reabsorbed from the ascending limb of Henle's loop, therefore the fluid entering the distal tubules is hypotonic with respect to the plasma. In the absence of ADH, the epithelium lining the distal tubules and collecting ducts is impermeable to water, and the urine remains hypotonic; in the presence of ADH, however, the epithelium becomes water-permeable, and water is osmotically extracted into the isotonic interstitium of the renal cortex. Under conditions of even greater antidiuresis, water is absorbed also from the collecting ducts into the hypertonic renal medulla, and the urine which reaches the renal pelvis is considerably more concentrated than the plasma (up to 1,200 mOs/l).

The hypertonicity of the renal medulla depends on the activity of the countercurrent multiplier formed by the loops of Henle and, perhaps, by the vasa recta. Some workers suggest that ADH may affect blood flow through the vasa recta and, by thus influencing the efficiency of the medullary countercurrent system, may affect the hypertonicity of the interstitial fluid around the collecting ducts.

ABNORMALITIES OF WATER BALANCE

The chief problem with water balance is conservation, because, even under favourable circumstances, there is an unavoidable water loss through the skin, from the lungs, and particularly from the kidneys, amounting to at least to 1½ l/day; and in a hot environment sweating may greatly increase this water loss (see Chapter 13). To achieve water balance intake must keep pace with water loss, therefore anything which impairs the body's water intake is likely to cause water depletion.

Water excess is unlikely to occur, except when the ability of the kidneys to excrete an increased water load is depressed by disease or excessive ADH activity (see below).

Water deficits have relatively little effect on the cardiovascular system because they are spread throughout the total body water; whereas cardiovascular function is dependent mainly on the intravascular pressures which reflect mainly the intravascular fluid volume (see Chapter 7).

Water excess

Water excess may occur when renal excretory function is depressed, as by intrinsic renal disease, or by the inappropriate secretion of ADH. Under normal circumstances the body can increase its free water clearance (see earlier) many times, and can thus cope even with an extremely large dietary water intake, such as, say, the rapid ingestion of 10 pints of beer.

Inappropriate ADH secretion causes the kidneys to retain water irrespective of the body's need. It occurs, for example, when an intracranial lesion irritates the supraoptico-hypophysial tract, or when excessive amounts of ADH are secreted by a neoplasm, commonly a bronchial carcinoma.* ADH secretion is stimulated also by reduction of e.c.f. volume, as accompanies sodium depletion (q.v.); under these circumstances the stimulatory effects of e.c.f. depletion overcome the inhibitory effects of the reduction of extracellular osmolarity which accompanies water retention.

An excess of water is distributed throughout the body's various fluid compartments—intracellular fluid, interstitial fluid and plasma—roughly in proportion to their relative sizes. Extracellular fluid dilution is relatively unimportant; but expansion of the intracellular compartment leads to cellular overhydration in various organs, particularly the brain, and to symptoms of 'water intoxication' with headache, nausea, vomiting, confusion, and even convulsions.

---

*In recent years it has been increasingly realized that a variety of malignant tumours may synthesize a variety of polypeptide hormones with a variety of physiological effects.

Water depletion

Water depletion is particularly likely to occur when fluid loss is increased as a result of impaired renal concentrating ability (see earlier). But it may occur also in the presence of normal renal function if the patient's thirst mechanism is impaired. Normally, water depletion causes intense thirst, and so induces an increased water intake; in a confused, or unconscious patient, however, the thirst mechanism may be inoperative, or the patient may have some local condition which prevents an increase of water intake, e.g. oesophageal stricture.

The concentrating power of the kidneys may be impaired by intrinsic renal disease, e.g. chronic nephritis. In severe renal failure (q.v.) the osmolarity of the urine becomes fixed at approximately the same value as the plasma—isosthenuria. The kidney is also unable to produce a concentrated urine when ADH secretion is depressed, as in pituitary diabetes insipidus, or when the renal tubules are unresponsive to ADH, as in nephrogenic diabetes insipidus.

Water depletion affects all the body fluid compartments, roughly in proportion to their relative sizes; but it is only when the deficit becomes severe that reduction of e.c.f. volume produces the clinical signs of hypovolaemia and dehydration. If water depletion is severe, the patient may become confused and disorientated, and ultimately comatose. The concentration of all plasma solutes is increased but, as with water excess, the haematocrit ratio of the peripheral blood remains normal because the plasma and i.c.f. are both equally affected.

SODIUM

PHYSIOLOGY

As is the case with water, the body is normally in sodium equilibrium. Dietary intake varies between 100 and 300 mmol/day, and is just balanced by sodium loss in the urine and, in warm environments, in the sweat. In a temperate climate the body has no compulsory sodium loss comparable to its obligatory water loss, therefore it is able, if necessary, to reduce sodium loss almost to zero and thus compensate for a severe restriction of dietary sodium intake, down to 10 mmol/day or less. In a hot climate, sweating is very considerably increased and sodium loss by this route may be as great as 500 mmol/day (see next chapter).

Renal handling of sodium (see also Chapter 7)
Sodium is filtered from the plasma by the renal glomeruli. The majority of this filtered sodium is then reabsorbed from the renal

tubules, so that less than 1 per cent is normally excreted in the urine.

Some five-sixths of the filtered sodium is normally removed by the proximal tubules; this process appears to be relatively constant, and not under hormonal control.* (It may, however, be decreased by osmotic diuresis, as in diabetes (q.v.), when water reabsorption is impaired by the presence of abnormal amounts of glucose in the tubular fluid.) In the distal tubules, sodium reabsorption is adjusted in accordance with the body's needs by changes in the plasma levels of aldosterone and other hormones. Sodium reabsorption at this site occurs in association with the movement of potassium and hydrogen ions in the opposite direction, so that increased distal sodium reabsorption is accompanied by increased potassium loss.

The stimulus for an alteration in the rate of renal sodium excretion is a change of e.c.f. volume, rather than a change in its sodium concentration (which affects predominantly ADH secretion). Depletion of e.c.f. volume increases the rate of aldosterone secretion from the adrenal cortex and, by enhancing the rate of sodium/potassium exchange across the distal tubular cells, causes sodium retention. The site of the receptors which detect such changes of e.c.f. volume is uncertain; it is known, however, that the renal juxtaglomerular apparatus is concerned with the control of aldosterone secretion via the renin-angio tensin system (see section on hypertension).

ABNORMALITIES OF SODIUM BALANCE

Extracellular fluid volume is governed by the amount of sodium which it contains, because, under normal circumstances, the osmolarity of this compartment is maintained within narrow limits by the ADH mechanism (see section on water balance). The maintainance of sodium balance is therefore important because changes in e.c.f. volume have important consequences on the cardiovascular system (see sections on shock and oedema).

The chief problem with water balance is conservation; with sodium balance it is excretion. Renal sodium-retaining ability is normally so good that it is not possible to develop serious sodium depletion as a result of inadequate sodium intake unless dietary restriction is accompanied by impaired renal function or abnormal sodium loss by other routes. But in the presence of impaired renal function it is readily possible for sodium intake to exceed output even on a normal diet.

---

*Recent work however suggests that this statement may not be entirely true—see standard texts.

Sodium depletion

Sodium loss depletes the entire e.c.f. compartment, both plasma and interstitial fluid. On a percentage basis, however, the depletion of the intravascular compartment is less severe because the plasma protein osmotic pressure holds fluid intravascularly at the expense of the interstitial fluid; the haemodynamic consequences of sodium depletion are thus somewhat mitigated.

Excessive sodium loss occurs with loss of plasma in haemorrhage and burns, and with loss of e.c.f., as accompanies excessive sweating, vomiting and diarrhoea. (The sodium concentration of gastric juice is relatively low—Fig. 22. However, the alkalosis which accompanies prolonged vomiting causes the kidneys to excrete large quantities of bicarbonate ions. These anions must, of course, be accompanied by equal amounts of sodium or other cation, thus leading to sodium depletion. But, see later section on pyloric stenosis.)

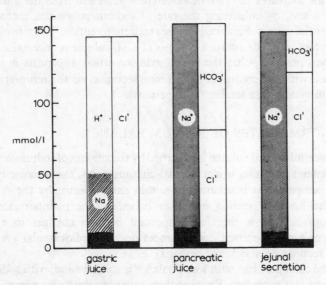

Fig. 22. Electrolyte composition of gastric juice, pancreatic juice and jejunal secretion.

Sodium depletion may occur also when there is renal malfunction. This may be the result of intrinsic renal disease, such as the diuretic phase of acute tubular necrosis (q.v.), or 'salt-losing nephritis' as a result of chronic pyelonephritis, or the result of inadequate hormonal control, as in Addison's disease. Excessive renal sodium loss also accompanies the osmotic diuresis of diabetic ketosis.

Reduction of e.c.f. volume by sodium depletion stimulates ADH secretion—probably via volume receptors in the left atrium—and thus reduces renal water loss. The depletion of e.c.f. volume is thereby reduced, although at the expense of its osmolarity and sodium concentration.

Depletion of the interstitial fluid compartment gives rise to the clinical signs of dehydration, with loss of skin elasticity and reduction of intraocular tension. If the depletion becomes severe there is reduction of cardiac filling pressure, and therefore of cardiac output (see Chapter 1). The body responds to such cardiovascular stress with vasoconstriction in a variety of organs, including the kidneys, causing depression of renal function and a rapid rise of blood urea concentration—the condition of pre-renal uraemia (see section on renal failure).

Sodium depletion may occur also as a result of heavy sweating. If the deficit of sodium and water is replaced by water only, the extracellular sodium concentration may be severely reduced resulting in painful muscular cramps—stokers'cramps.

Sodium retention

Sodium retention expands both compartments of the e.c.f., thus causing an increase of cardiac output and a generalized tendency to oedema formation (see below). It occurs whenever dietary sodium intake exceeds renal excretory ability. It may thus accompany intrinsic renal disease, and abnormalities of renal function due to disease elsewhere in the body, as when renal perfusion is decreased by chronic heart failure, and when sodium reabsorption is enhanced by increased aldosterone activity.

(Note, however, that excessive aldosterone production by a glomerulosa-cell tumour of the adrenal cortex—primary hyperaldosteronism, Conn's syndrome—seldom gives rise to oedema, unless there is concomitant heart failure as a result of the systemic hypertension which accompanies this condition.)

When the plasma proteins are reduced in amount, plasma volume is reduced also, roughly in proportion to the size of the protein deficit. This situation may occur, for example, when there is defective albumin formation in hepatic disease, or when there is excessive protein loss in the nephrotic syndrome, or in protein-losing enteropathy. The resulting hypovolaemia stimulates aldosterone secretion, probably via the renin-angiotensin mechanism (see section on hypertension), and thus induces sodium retention with consequent expansion of the e.c.f. compartment and development of oedema. Expansion of the intravascular compartment in this way ameliorates the patient's hypovolaemia thereby preventing the fall of cardiac output which would otherwise occur.

(The above paragraph probably does not tell the whole story, however, because the sodium retention which characterizes hypoproteinaemic states is not usually associated with excessive urinary potassium loss, as would be the case if it was due solely to the action of aldosterone on the distal tubules. There is evidence that the sodium retention of hypoproteinaemia is due chiefly to increased sodium reabsorption from the proximal tubules, which are usually assumed not to be influenced by aldosterone.)

OEDEMA

PHYSIOLOGY

There is a constant exchange of cystalloid-containing fluid across the capillary membrane which separates the intravascular and extravascular compartments; fluid moves out at the arterial end of the capillary, and back in again at its venous end. Oedema occurs when this fluid exchange is deranged, and may result either from a local abnormality or from a generalized expansion of the e.c.f., as accompanies sodium retention (see above). Clinically, oedema is said to occur when the interstitial fluid volume is expanded by more than about 10 per cent of its normal size.

The intravascular pressure at the arterial end of a capillary is approximately 30 mmHg. This pressure exceeds the colloid osmotic pressure (oncotic pressure) of the plasma proteins (about 25 mmHg), therefore fluid is forced out of the capillary into the interstitial fluid compartment. At the venous end of the capillary, the intravascular pressure is only about 10 mmHg, while the protein oncotic pressure is the same (or somewhat increased by the loss of fluid which occurs at the arterial end); interstitial fluid therefore returns to the intravascular compartment, leaving only a small amount to be carried away by the lymphatics.

(Recent research suggests that the pressure in the interstitial fluid compartment is sub-atmospheric ('negative'), a factor which aids filtration out of the capillaries.)

The fact that, in most tissues, lymph contains a certain amount of protein indicates that, contrary to what is often assumed, the capillary membrane is *not* completely impermeable to large molecules. This lymphatic protein concentration varies from tissue to tissue, suggesting that the permeability of the capillary membrane varies also; it is particularly high in the liver, spleen and bone marrow, a finding which may be related to the fact that these organs do not have true capillaries, but sinusoids lined with reticuloendothelial cells.

PATHOGENESIS OF OEDEMA

A knowledge of physiology suggests that oedema should occur in the following situations: when the intracapillary pressure is raised, when the plasma protein concentration is reduced, when lymphatic drainage is impeded, when capillary permeability is increased by inflammation or allergy, and when there is generalized e.c.f. expansion, secondary to sodium retention. This does, in fact, appear to be the case.

Increase of intracapillary pressure occurs as a result of generalized venous congestion, e.g. in chronic heart failure, or as a result of local venous obstruction from thrombosis, etc. It accompanies also the arteriolar dilatation of inflammation (see below). (It is now thought that the oedema of heart failure occurs chiefly as the result of sodium retention from defective renal function, i.e. from 'forward' rather than 'backward' failure—see section on heart failure.)

Plasma protein concentration is reduced in the nephrotic syndrome, in chronic hepatic failure (q.v.) and in protein-losing enteropathy. The nephrotic syndrome is characterized by excessive loss of protein in the urine. It may arise in a variety of ways, including renal vein thrombosis (rare), poisoning with heavy metals or drugs, amyloid disease and, most commonly, primary renal disease, in which there is increased protein permeability of the glomerular capillaries. In this condition, and in protein-losing enteropathy, protein is lost from the body faster than it can be resynthetized in the liver. In hepatic failure, protein synthesis is impaired, and the body is consequently unable to make good its normal protein catabolism. As explained earlier, reduction in the total amount of protein present in the plasma stimulates aldosterone secretion from the adrenal cortex, and thus aggravates the already-present tendency to oedema formation.

Of the plasma proteins, albumin is osmotically the more important. Not only is it normally present in the greatest concentration (45 g/l, cf. globulin 25 g/l and fibrinogen 3 g/l), but its molecular weight (68 000) is much less than that of either globulin or fibrinogen. Thus some five-sixths of the normal plasma oncotic pressure is due to albumin. It is of course the smaller molecules which are preferentially lost from the circulation when there is increased capillary permeability.

Lymphatic obstruction causes local oedema, as when the lymphatics are obstructed by a neoplasm, or by postinflammatory fibrosis as in filariasis (elephantiasis).

The oedema which surrounds an area of inflammation is due not only to increased capillary intravascular pressure, consequent on arteriolar dilatation, but also to capillary wall damage by the inflammatory or allergic process. Such damage permits protein to leak out into the interstitial space, where, by raising the local colloid osmotic pressure, it encourages oedema formation.

The causes of generalized sodium retention have already been considered (see earlier).

POTASSIUM

PHYSIOLOGY

Normally, the potassium which appears in the glomerular filtrate is completely reabsorbed before the end of the proximal convoluted tubules. The potassium which is excreted in the urine has been resecreted into the distal tubules. This process involves the exchange of sodium and potassium ions across the tubular endothelium, a process which is enhanced by aldosterone, and by an increase in the amount of sodium reaching the distal tubules, as happens in osmotic diuresis and after the administration of certain diuretics.

Sodium ions also exchange with hydrogen ions across the walls of the distal tubules. This process occurs in competition with the sodium/potassium exchange mentioned in the previous paragraph, therefore potassium and hydrogen ion excretion tend to be reciprocally related. In alkalosis, hydrogen ions are present in reduced amounts, potassium excretion is thereby enhanced: conversely, in the presence of potassium deficiency, excessive amounts of hydrogen ions are lost in the urine, causing a metabolic alkalosis.

A rather similar relationship exists between the exchange of potassium and hydrogen ions across cell membranes generally. Potassium deficiency depletes the intracellular cations; hydrogen (and sodium) ions therefore move into the cells, causing an intracellular acidosis and an extracellular alkalosis. (The respiratory response to this situation is, of course, dependent mainly on the intracellular, rather than the extracellular, hydrogen ion concentration; it therefore tends to be paradoxical.)

ABNORMALITIES OF POTASSIUM BALANCE

Potassium balance is relatively independent of the body's sodium and water content, but is intimately related to its acid-base state (see section on pyloric stenosis). The majority of the body's potassium is located in its intracellular compartment (see Fig. 20). As a result, the diagnosis of abnormalities of potassium balance may be very difficult, because analysis of e.c.f., as represented by the plasma, does not necessarily reveal the ionic composition of the i.c.f.; and considerable reliance must be placed on the patient's history, and on the clinician's knowledge of the circumstances under which abnormalities of potassium balance may occur.

Potassium depletion

Renal potassium conservation is considerably less well developed than is the case with sodium. Potassium depletion may thus occur as a result of dietary restriction, as in anorexia, or when intravenous feeding with non-potassium-containing fluids is unduly prolonged. Severe depletion of this cation, however, usually means that there has been abnormal potassium loss from the gastrointestinal tract, or in the urine.

Gastric juice contains only some 5 mmol/l of potassium (the same concentration as in plasma), therefore the potassium deficiency which accompanies severe vomiting is not due solely, or even mainly, to loss of potassium in the vomitus. However, there is in this condition increased aldosterone secretion as a result of e.c.f. depletion, and therefore a considerable loss of potassium in the urine (see section on pyloric stenosis). Also, the alkalosis which accompanies prolonged vomiting tends to promote potassium transfer across the distal tubular cells, thus aggravating potassium loss.

The concentrations of sodium and potassium in the secretions of the upper gastrointestinal tract are approximately the same as those in e.c.f. (see Fig. 22). In the distal intestine, however, the sodium:potassium ratio is approximately 1:2, therefore excessive loss of lower intestinal contents as in diarrhoea is particularly likely to cause potassium deficiency.

The clinical manifestations of potassium deficiency are relatively non-specific; and it is thus necessary to consider the possibility of this condition whenever potassium intake is severely reduced, or when there is increased potassium loss by any route. Intracellular potassium deficiency may not be reflected in the composition of the extracellular fluid, although there may be a movement of sodium and hydrogen ions intracellularly to compensate for the loss of intracellular potassium; these ionic movements may be reflected in hyponatraemia and alkalosis in the plasma.

Potassium deficiency is commonly accompanied by mental symptoms, such as apathy, loss of memory and confusion. There is also impairment of the contractility of all types of muscle—smooth, cardiac and skeletal—with weakness of the peripheral muscles, leading ultimately to flaccid paralysis with loss of the deep tendon reflexes, abdominal distension and even paralytic ileus, and impaired myocardial contractility and arterial hypotension.

The poor cardiac function is accompanied by electrocardiographic changes, with small T waves, QT prolongation, ST segment depression and U waves. Potassium deficiency also increases the susceptibility of the heart to digitalis glycosides—a point to be considered in the treatment of congestive cardiac failure with diuretics.

Magnesium deficiency

Magnesium deficiency is likely to occur in the same circumstances as potassium deficiency, and may be accompanied by very similar non-specific manifestations. This condition is being increasingly recognized, and should be looked for whenever there is a possibility of potassium deficiency (see section on pyloric stenosis).

Potassium retention

In the presence of normal renal function it is impossible to cause hyperkalaemia by oral potassium administration, although this condition can, of course, be iatrogenically produced by the rapid intravenous administration of large amounts of potassium salts. In the presence of anuria or severe oliguria, i.e. with acute renal failure or in the terminal stages of chronic renal failure however, potassium retention is a common occurrence, and the resulting hyperkalaemia can, and commonly does, lead to fatal ventricular fibrillation. This is particularly likely to occur when there is increased cellular breakdown, permitting intracellular potassium ions to move into the plasma.

A raised plasma potassium concentration is accompanied by characteristic e.c.g. changes, with tenting of the T waves, ST segment depression, flattening of the P waves, and prolongation of the QRS complex, rather like that seen in bundle-branch block—see Figure 23.

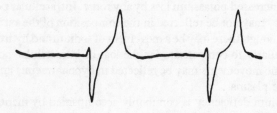

Fig. 23. Electrocardiogram in extreme hyperkalaemia (courtesty of Dr A. C. F. Kenmure).

ACID-BASE BALANCE

PHYSIOLOGY

Students—and others—traditionally find acid-base balance difficult and esoteric; but, given a basic understanding of the terminology, it is in fact no more difficult to understand than any other aspect of physiology.

Acid-base balance has to do with the concentration of hydrogen ions, $[H^+]$, in the body fluids. In practice this means in the e.c.f., because (as with potassium) it is difficult to measure intracellular $[H^+]$. To function efficiently the body's cells must be provided with an environment in which the $[H^+]$ is maintained within certain limits. And, just as is the case with other ions, there are factors which tend to shift the $[H^+]$ outside the normal range, and homeostatic mechanisms which resist these changes.

Following a meal, hydrocholoric acid is secreted into the stomach, leaving the blood relatively alkaline ($[H^+]$ decreased); later bicarbonate-containing pancreatic fluid is secreted into the duodenum, restoring the plasma $[H^+]$ towards normal. The result is the well-known postprandial alkaline tide. Severe exercise is accompanied by the production of large amounts of lactic acid in the exercising muscles (see section on metabolic acidosis). Also, the level of arterial P_{CO_2} (and therefore $[H^+]$—see later) varies in response to the changes of pulmonary ventilation which accompany speech, and the hyperventilation of emotional excitement and mild or moderate exercise. In all these cases the resulting $[H^+]$ changes are minimized by various buffers (see below).

In disease, the forces tending to disturb acid-base balance may be so great that the body's homeostatic mechanisms are overwhelmed; the result is acidosis or alkalosis.

Terminology

An acid is a substance which can dissociate to give rise to (donate) hydrogen ions; a base is a substance which accepts hydrogen ions. Thus:

$$HA \rightleftharpoons H^+ + A'$$
$$\text{acid} \qquad \text{base}$$

Typical acids in the body are hydrochloric, carbonic and lactic acid; typical bases are bicarbonate ions, chloride ions, and ammonia (in the renal tubules).

Certain ions can act both as acids and as bases. Thus, proteins can donate hydrogen ions by ionization of their COOH groups, or accept hydrogen ions by combining these with their NH_2 groups. In an alkaline environment (where hydrogen ions are deficient) the first reaction predominates: in an acid environment the second.

Substances which are only partially dissociated into hydrogen ions can act as *buffers*, i.e. as substances which can limit changes in $[H^+]$. When an acid is added to a buffer solution the added hydrogen ions combine with the buffer ions to form undissociated buffer; conversely, when hydrogen ions are removed from the buffer solution the undissociated buffer donates hydrogen ions, and thereby limits the $[H^+]$ change.

A buffer is most effective when it is half dissociated. The $[H^+]$ at which this is so depends on the particular buffer under consideration. One of the most important buffers in the body is protein, particularly haemoglobin. Proteins contain COOH and NH_2 groups, both of which can act as buffers (see above); but at the normal $[H^+]$ of the body fluids these groups tend to be either fully dissociated (COO') or fully associated (NH_3^+), and therefore have little buffering power. Proteins however also contain imidazole groups, which can also act as buffers, and being roughly halfway dissociated at the normal body $[H^+]$, can do so very effectively. Imidazole groups are particularly numerous in the protein moiety of haemoglobin.

Haemoglobin has another important property which enhances its *in vivo* buffering capacity. When haemoglobin becomes reduced, as in the peripheral tissues, its tendency to accept hydrogen ions is increased, i.e. it becomes a weaker acid and is therefore better able to mop up hydrogen ions produced by tissue metabolism.

pH

It is not in fact usual to speak about the hydrogen ion concentration of the body fluids, but rather about their pH. There are certain theoretical reasons for this convention; but these are not important here, and it is best to regard the use of the pH notation as a slightly awkward historical hangover.

pH is defined as $-\log_{10} [H^+]$, where $[H^+]$ is the hydrogen ion concentration (or strictly hydrogen ion activity). From this formula it is possible to draw up a conversion table:

pH	$[H^+]$
7.0	100 nmol/l
7.4	40 nmol/l
8.0	10 nmol/l

And, since the range of blood pH which is compatible with life is approximately 6.8 to 7.8, it can be seen that, far from being controlled within very narrow limits as is often stated, the range of [H⁺] found in life may be rather large, cf. other ions such as sodium and calcium. (Remember, however, that we have very little information about the range of intracellular pH.)

METABOLIC AND RESPIRATORY ACID-BASE DISTURBANCES

It is usual—and convenient, since the pathogenesis and treatment of the two conditions is very different—to separate acid-base disturbances into two broad categories: respiratory and metabolic. The former are due to abnormalities in the partial pressure (tension) of carbon dioxide in the blood,* the latter to abnormalities in the amounts of other acids. (The use of the term metabolic in this context is illogical: one of the chief products of metabolism is carbon dioxide, which by definition is not included in a consideration of metabolic acid-base disturbances; a better term, which is unfortunately not in general use, is non-respiratory acid-base disturbance.)

Respiratory acidosis and alkalosis
As explained in Chapter 4 anything which depresses the level of alveolar ventilation in relation to the body's metabolic carbon dioxide production causes an increase in the partial pressure of carbon dioxide in the arterial blood. This is accompanied by an increase in plasma [H⁺] according to the equation:

$$CO_2 + H_2O \rightleftharpoons H^+ + HCO'_3$$

This is the condition of respiratory acidosis which is considered further in the section on ventilatory failure (q.v.).

The converse condition of respiratory alkalosis is due to increased alveolar ventilation. It occurs in salicylate poisoning (probably from a direct stimulatory effect on the respiratory centre), with intense emotional stimulation, e.g. fear of visiting the dentist, and in hysterical over-breathing. In the latter two conditions the resulting alkalosis may depress the level of ionized calcium in the blood sufficiently to cause overt or latent tetany (see section on calcium).

Respiratory acid-base changes are accompanied by changes in renal H⁺ excretion (see section on respiratory failure and Chapter 7). These

---

*Carbon dioxide combines with water to form carbonic acid which dissociates to produce hydrogen ions; it may therefore be regarded as an acid.

compensatory changes restore the blood pH to, or towards, normal. A respiratory acidosis is accompanied by a compensatory metabolic alkalosis: a respiratory alkalosis is accompanied by a compensatory metabolic acidosis (see below).

Metabolic acidosis and alkalosis

Metabolic acid-base disturbances occur when there is abnormal loss of gastrointestinal contents. In vomiting, for example, there is a predominant loss of acid, resulting in a metabolic alkalosis; in diarrhoea there is a predominant loss of base (bicarbonate), resulting in a metabolic acidosis.

Metabolic acidosis occurs also after a cardiac arrest. Tissue metabolism is normally aerobic, i.e. energy is liberated by the aerobic breakdown of various substrates to carbon dioxide and water. But when there is an absolute or relative deficiency of oxygen the tissues must derive all or part of their metabolic energy requirements from the anaerobic breakdown of glucose to lactic acid. The accumulation of this acid in the peripheral blood causes a metabolic acidosis. This is the situation during a cardiac arrest; and particularly so when tissue perfusion is restored after a period of circulatory arrest or severe inadequacy, when lactic acid, formed in the ischaemic tissues, is washed out into the general circulation.

A similar situation occurs during heavy exercise. In this case cardiac output, although greatly above normal, is still insufficient to supply oxygen to the exercising tissues fast enough for them to be able to derive all the energy they require from aerobic metabolism.

A metabolic acidosis stimulates the respiratory centre(s) and causes an increase of pulmonary ventilation, thus inducing a (compensatory) respiratory alkalosis and partial restoration of the blood pH. A metabolic alkalosis is similarly accompanied by a compensatory respiratory acidosis.

QUANTIFICATION OF ACID-BASE DISTURBANCES

To assess the severity of a respiratory acid-base disturbance is simple. The normal arterial P_{CO_2} is 40 mmHg: a value above this is a respiratory acidosis; a value below it is a respiratory alkalosis. And the severity of the disturbance is given by the extent to which the P_aCO_2 departs from the normal 40 mmHg.

The situation in the case of a metabolic disturbance is, however, more difficult. Addition of a strong acid e.g. lactic acid to the blood reduces the concentration of bicarbonate ions, thereby pushing the reaction to the right; the removal of hydrogen ions pushes it to the left. A metabolic acidosis is therefore accompanied by a reduction in the plasma [HCO'_3], a metabolic alkalosis by an increase in plasma [HCO'_3]. It might be thought therefore that it would be a simple matter to quantify the severity of a patient's metabolic acid-base disturbance by measuring his plasma bicarbonate ion concentration. Unfortunately this is not the case, because changes in P_{CO_2} (respiratory acid-base disturbances) themselves alter the plasma [HCO'_3], also according to the above equation. (A respiratory acidosis, for example, is accompanied by an increase in [HCO'_3]). Therefore an abnormal plasma bicarbonate concentration may indicate *either* a metabolic acid-base disturbance, *or* a respiratory acid-base disturbance, or *both* together.

$$HCO'_3 + H^+ \rightleftharpoons H_2O + CO_2$$

The way round this difficulty is, in fact, simple. A sample of blood is taken from the patient and artificially brought to the normal P_{CO_2} of 40 mmHg; the bicarbonate concentration is measured, and compared with the normal value of 21 to 25 mmol/l. The bicarbonate concentration so measured,* i.e. at a P_{CO_2} of 40 mmHg—and at a temperature of 37°C, with the blood fully oxygenated—is called the *standard* bicarbonate concentration. It is then readily possible to see if the patient has a metabolic acid-base disturbance, because the effects of any super-added respiratory disturbance have been eliminated.

A standard bicarbonate concentration below the normal range indicates a metabolic acidosis; a value above this range indicates a metabolic alkalosis. And the severity of the disturbance is given by the magnitude of the departure from normality.

(It is also possible to assess the severity of a patient's metabolic acid-base disturbance by calculating, from the pH and P_{CO_2} of his blood, his so-called *base excess*. This is the amount of acid (mmol/l) which would have to be added to the blood to restore its acid-base state to normal, i.e. to a P_{CO_2} of 40 mmHg, and a pH of 7.40. The normal value of base excess is, of course, approximately zero: in metabolic alkalosis it is positive; in metabolic acidosis it is negative.)

It is common practice to represent acid-base disturbances graphically on diagrams such as the Siggaard-Andersen nomogram, or the Davenport diagram. Examples of the use of these are given on pages 49 and 89—for further details see any of the standard undergraduate physiology texts.

---

*In practice the concentration is usually calculated rather than measured.

MIXED ELECTROLYTE ABNORMALITIES

For descriptive purposes it is convenient to consider single electrolyte abnormalities in isolation. But this is not, of course, how such conditions present clinically. Here mixed abnormalities are the rule; and isolated defects of the type considered earlier are uncommon.

It is obviously not possible here to deal in detail with all the many known electrolyte imbalance syndromes; but a study of one such condition—chronic pyloric stenosis—gives valuable insight into the way in which abnormalities of water, sodium, potassium and acid-base balance can interact to produce what must inevitably be a somewhat complicated picture.

Chronic pyloric stenosis

Chronic obstruction of the pylorus from peptic ulceration is a relatively common condition. It is a mechanical lesion which prevents the entry of gastric contents into the small intestine; and it is therefore accompanied by vomiting, and considerable fluid and electrolyte loss. The late end results of neglected pyloric obstruction (as considered here) are fortunately seldom seen in medically-advanced countries; but they do occur.

Initially the vomiting causes loss of water, hydrochloric acid, and of sodium, potassium and chloride ions. (The relative amount of these constituents varies somewhat from patient to patient.) And, since the secretion of each hydrogen ion into the stomach is accompanied by the passage of one bicarbonate ion into the plasma, the loss of gastric contents is accompanied by an increase in plasma $[HCO'_3]$, i.e. by a metabolic alkalosis (usually with a slight respiratory compensation—see earlier).

At this time, early in the course of the disease, the urine is alkaline, and contains an excess of bicarbonate ions as the kidneys try to restore the body's acid-base balance. There is also increased renal sodium loss (because sodium ions accompany bicarbonate ions lost in the urine) with aggravation of the e.c.f. depletion caused by the vomiting. In early, mild cases this extracellular fluid depletion is not clinically apparent; but as it progresses it becomes so, and stimulates aldosterone secretion from the adrenal cortex (see section on sodium balance), and thus enhances sodium/potassium exchange across the walls of the distal convoluted tubules.

Sodium therefore disappears almost completely from the urine; and renal potassium loss accentuates the pre-existing potassium loss in the vomitus, giving rise to a marked potassium depletion (q.v.). There is thus hypokalaemia with clinical signs of potassium depletion. The blood sodium concentration remains relatively normal.

The increased aldosterone activity also causes increased sodium /hydrogen ion exchange in the distal tubules. There is therefore increased loss of hydrogen ions in the urine, which paradoxically becomes *acid*, even though the blood continues to exhibit a considerable metabolic alkalosis. In addition, there is an increased movement of sodium ions into the cells, and a movement of potassium ions in the opposite direction, thus tending to maintain the plasma potassium concentration. Hydrogen ions also move intracellularly, accentuating the extracellular alkalosis, and causing an intracellular acidosis.

The patient is now very ill, with clinical evidence of severe dehydration, and of hypokalaemia with mental confusion and muscular weakness—see section on potassium deficiency. Biochemically he has a (partially compensated) metabolic alkalosis with a severe reduction of plasma chloride concentration, a marked reduction of plasma standard bicarbonate concentration, a lesser reduction of plasma potassium concentration, and a relatively normal plasma sodium concentration; the urine is acid. The degree of alkalosis may be sufficiently severe for the patient to develop tetany.

In neglected cases the reduction of e.c.f. volume may be sufficient to cause peripheral circulatory failure (q.v.) with reduction of renal blood flow and the development of pre-renal uraemia (see section on renal failure). This situation is aggravated by the fact that the patient's oral intake of energy ('calories') is so reduced that he derives most of his energy requirements from the metabolism of his own tissues, thus increasing the excretory load on the kidneys.

Treatment

The basic lesion in pyloric stenosis is mechanical, and obviously can be relieved only by mechanical means, i.e. by operation. Before this can be done, however, the patient must be got into a condition to withstand a fairly major surgical procedure.

Opinions differ on the best emergency treatment of a patient with severe pyloric stenosis as described above. On the one hand, there are those who say that the intravenous infusion of adequate amounts of isotonic sodium chloride solution (9 g/l), plus suitable potassium supplements (e.g. 1 or 2 g/l of intravenous fluid) will restore renal function to the point where the patient's kidneys can take over the fine adjustment of his biochemical state. On the other hand there are those who think that the clinician should attempt to reverse each and every biochemical abnormality e.g. by the infusion of ammonium chloride solution to reverse the patient's alkalosis, and so on. Probably the former approach is nearer to the ideal than the latter.

FURTHER READING

Anon 1977 Natriuretic hormone. Lancet, ii: 537

Anon 1978 Hyponatraemia Lancet i 642

Anon 1979 Exercise oedema Lancet i 961

Black D A K 1976 Essential of Fluid Balance, 4th edn. Oxford: Blackwell.

Campbell E J M 1962 RIpH. Lancet i: 681

Campbell E J M Dickinson C J & Slater J D H 1974 Clinical Physiology 4th edn, chap. 1. Oxford: Blackwell

Cattell, W R 1967 The physiological basis of fluid and electrolyte balance. British Journal of Hospital Medicine 1, 1130

Cattell W R 1968 The assessment and management of fluid and electrolyte balance. British Journal of Hospital Medicine 2: 419

Committee of New York Academy of Sciences Conference. 1965 Acid-base terminology. Lancet, ii: 1010

Davenport, H W 1970 The ABC of Acid-base Chemistry, 5th edn. University of Chicago Press

Flenley D C 1971 Another non-logarithmic acid-base diagram? Lancet i: 961

Gamble J L 1954 Chemical Anatomy, Physiology and Pathology of Extracellular Fluid, 6th edn. Cambridge, Mass.: Harvard University Press

Goldberger E 1970 A Primer of Water, Electrolyte and Acid-base Syndromes, 4th edn. Philadelphia: Lea & Febiger

Hoffman W S 1970 The Biochemistry of Clinical Medicine, 4th edn, chap. 6. Chicago: Year Book Medical Publishers

Lever A F 1965 The vasa recta and countercurrent multiplication. Acta medica scandinavica 178: suppl. 434: 1

Robinson J R 1972 Fundamentals of Acid-base Regulation 4th edn. London: Blackwell

Wilkinson A W 1973 Body Fluids in Surgery. Edinburgh and London: Churchill Livingstone

13

Hypothermia and hyperthermia

Despite wide environmental temperature variations, man maintains his deep-body temperature constant to better than a°C by a variety of physiological and behavioural responses. Failure of these homeostatic mechanisms may lead to the pathological state of hypothermia, or the (much less common) condition of hyperthermia or hyperpyrexia. A naked human requires a surrounding air temperature of about 28°C if he is to maintain thermal balance. This is of course much higher than the environmental temperatures which are normally found in temperate climates*; and it is usual to raise artificially the temperature of the air immediately adjacent to the skin (the body's 'microclimate') by wearing clothes, and by living in artificially heated dwellings.

In addition, the body is able to compensate for small changes in external temperature by varying the effective thickness of its peripheral insulating layer (see Fig 24) by changes of vascular sympathetic nervous activity; but the ability of these vascular mechanisms to keep the deep-body temperature constant is limited, and the body has other more powerful mechanisms which come into play if the temperature departs by more than a degree or so from the optimum 36° to 37°C. An increase of body temperature is accompanied by sweating, which increases heat loss from the body surface by evaporation of water; a decrease of body temperature is accompanied by an involuntary increase of heat production in the form of shivering. Both these mechanisms place a severe burden on the economy of the body (see below), and must therefore be regarded as second-line defences against changes of body temperature.

Of the two mechanisms the ability of the body to lower its temperature by increased secretion of sweat is the more powerful, and hot environments are consequently better tolerated than cold ones: clinically hypothermia is much more common than hyperthermia.

*Man probably evolved in the tropics where environmental temperatures of 28°C are of course common.

It is now well recognized that hypothermia is a constant danger whenever people are exposed to wet-cold conditions*, e.g. hill-walking, sailing, diving and deep sea fishing. In addition, it is now becoming increasingly recognized that minor degrees of hypothermia are very common in the elderly, and to a less extent in the new-born. It has, for example, been estimated—perhaps on not very good evidence—that as many as 20 000 old people die each year from hypothermia; and it is thought that mild degrees of hypothermia may contribute to the high accident rates which are found in the construction, deep sea fishing and diving industries.

PHYSIOLOGY

In common with other mammals, and birds, man maintains an almost constant deep-body temperature, i.e. is a homeotherm. This adaptation is advantageous in that it permits the body's vital organs to function with optimal efficiency, whatever—within reason—the environmental conditions; but at the same time it carries a penalty because maintenance of a constant body temperature in adverse conditions involves the expenditure of energy to produce heat, or the loss of large quantities of salt and water in sweat.

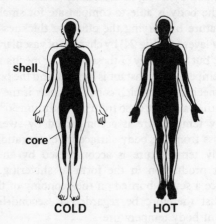

shell

core

COLD   HOT

Fig. 24. Variation of thickness of peripheral insulating "shell" in different thermal environments.

*The thermal insulation of ordinary clothing depends almost exclusively on air trapped in the interstices of the material. If this air is replaced by water the insulating value of the clothing falls almost to zero, i.e. the wearer is thermally naked.

The maintenance of a constant temperature requires a balance between the rate at which heat is produced by (or is added to) the body and the rate at which heat is lost to the environment. This thermal balance is achieved by surrounding the body's central tissues—its 'core' (see below)—with a peripheral 'shell' of tissue which does *not* have a constant temperature, and which acts as a variable insulator between the body's central core and its external environment (Fig. 24). Changes in the insulating value of the body's peripheral shell are brought about by changes in its blood supply as a result of changes in sympathetic nervous activity (see below, and p. 17). In addition, the body has mechanisms for involuntarily increasing its heat production by shivering when peripheral vasoconstriction is insufficient to maintain thermal balance in the cold, and mechanisms for increasing its rate of heat loss by sweating when peripheral vasodilation is insufficient to compensate for a hot environment. Also, man can of course aid these homeostatic mechanisms by behavioural responses, such as wearing appropriate clothing and living in airconditioned buildings.

Body temperature

The core temperature

The normal deep-body temperature is usually taken to be 37°C or 98.4°F. But there is in fact a consistent diurnal temperature variation of about 0.5°C (see below); and the deep-body temperature varies slightly from one core region to another. Wherever it is measured the body's core temperature is lowest in the early morning, and highest in the late afternoon or early evening, a typical variation (oral temperature) being from 36°C in the morning to 36.5°C in the evening.

This diurnal ('circadian') variation is to some extent the result of diurnal variations of food intake and physical activity; but it is still seen when experimental subjects are confined to bed and fed uniform meals at regular intervals; a finding which suggests that the body's metabolism is regulated also by an (unidentified) internal 'clock'. (There is at the present time considerable interest in the general subject of circadian rhythms, which affect not only body temperature, but also a variety of other bodily functions including: hormone secretion, appetite, urinary output of water and electrolytes, therapeutic response to various drugs and mental performance. A knowledge of these circadian variations is important for an understanding of the phenomenon of 'jet lag', in which rapid movement across several time-zones results in asynchrony between the body's internal clock and its external environment.)

In addition, there is a small monthly temperature variation in ovulating females, with a rise of up to 0.5°C at about the time of ovulation. This rise is thought to be due to increased circulating concentrations of progesterone, and may be useful for indicating the occurrence and timing of ovulation.

The peripheral temperature

In contrast to the relative constancy of the body's core temperature, the temperature of its skin and superficial tissues varies widely from region to region, and particularly with the body's need to lose or conserve heat. The skin temperature tends to be higher centrally than peripherally; and this is particularly so when there is peripheral vasoconstriction, as happens when the body needs to conserve heat in a cold environment (see Fig. 24). The average skin temperature of an individual who feels comfortably warm is around 33°C.

Heat gain

The body has a minimal rate of heat production due to its basal metabolism, that is the metabolic processes which maintain the resting function of the heart, lungs, brain etc. This basal heat production is supplemented by heat produced as a result of muscular activity, and by the so-called 'specific dynamic action' of ingested food. The normal basal heat production is about 170kJ/hr (40Cal/hr) per square metre body surface in the male, and rather less in the female. This amounts to a heat load of approximately 7.3 MJ (1700 Cal) which has to be dissipated to maintain the body in thermal balance. In the absence of external heat loss the body's basal heat production would result in an increase of body temperature of about 1°C/hr.

Normally of course heat production considerably exceeds the basal values given above—a typical 24 hour heat production would be 12 MJ (3000 Cal) in a sedentary worker, and perhaps as high as 18 MJ (4500 Cal) in a heavy manual worker. And during short periods of intense physical activity the body produces large amounts of heat in a short time, causing an increase of deep-body temperature of one or two degrees.

Exposure to cold results in an increase of body heat production, both voluntary and involuntary. There is for example a marked increase of muscular activity (stamping etc), which is in marked contrast to the decreased physical activity which is characteristic of hot environments, particularly during the heat of the day. In addition, exposure to cold causes an increase in *in*voluntary heat production, both in the form of shivering and as a hormonally-induced increase in body metabolism (non-shivering thermogenesis), although the importance of this latter response in man is disputed.

(Infants have deposits of specialized adipose tissue—brown fat—between their shoulder blades. This tissue is metabolically much more active than ordinary fat, and can produce large quantities of heat in response to sympathetic stimulation. In man these fat deposits atrophy with increasing age; but in hibernating animals the brown fat does not disappear, and plays an important role in increasing the animal's heat production after hibernation.)

Normally heat is lost from the body surface to the environment (see below), but heat transfer may occur also in the opposite direction, for example when the body is exposed to intense sunlight. This is why, for example, it is possible in bright sunshine to ski comfortably wearing relatively light clothing, even when the surrounding air temperature is below freezing. In a hot climate the amount of heat which can be added to the body by absorption of solar radiation is considerable, and may easily overwhelm the body's ability to maintain thermal balance (see below).

Heat loss

Heat loss from the body occurs mainly from the skin and lungs, and to a much less extent in the urine and faeces. Some of this heat loss is unavoidable, some is under the control of the body's thermoregulatory mechanisms.

The rate of loss depends on the extent to which the body is thermally insulated from its environment, and on the environmental conditions. In a temperate climate the environment is normally below 37°C, and heat is lost from the body surface by the physical processes of conduction, convection, evaporation, and radiation (convection being the most important); but when the environmental temperature is above body temperature the tendency is to *gain* heat from the environment by conduction and radiation. Under these circumstances the *only* way in which the body can lose heat is by evaporation of water from the lungs and body surface; if the environmental humidity is high this evaporation cannot occur, and the person is in danger of developing hyperthermia or 'heat stroke' (see later).

Convective heat loss from the 'body surface' is considerably enhanced by air movement, a fact which explains the chilling effect of a cold wind—'wind-chill'.

Heat loss by the evaporation of water takes place from the lungs and from the skin, even in the absence of obvious sweat production. Expired air is saturated with water vapour which represents a loss of about 500 ml of water daily (see p. 87); a similar loss occurs through the skin—insensible perspiration. The body has no means of regulating either of these sources of insensible water loss, although their magnitude is influenced by atmospheric conditions, particularly the relative humidity.

Since the evaporation of 1 g of water requires about 2.4 kJ (0.6 Cal) of latent heat, the loss of 1 l of water from the lungs and as insensible perspiration results in the loss of about 2.4 MJ (600 Cal) of heat per day, i.e. about 20 per cent of the body's resting heat production. In the presence of marked sweating, evaporative heat loss may be very considerable (see below).

The rate of cutaneous heat loss is modified by voluntarily adjusting the amount of clothing worn, and by reflex alterations in the vascularity of the body's peripheral insulating shell. However, even when the peripheral tissues are maximally vasodilated, the body's subcutaneous fat layer still provides some degree of thermal insulation, amounting to about 0.3 Clo (see below) in a person of average build. Air movement reduces the insulating value of ordinary clothing considerably, because most of its thermal insulation is provided by air trapped inside the interstices of the material: wind disturbs this trapped air, and so increases convective heat loss.

It is possible to quantify the insulating value of different types of clothing in terms of so-called Clo units. One Clo is the thermal insulation provided by an ordinary light-weight business suit, or the equivalent clothing in the case of a female, and permits the maintenance of a comfortable skin temperature (about 33°C) when the wearer is sitting at rest with an air temperature of 21°C and only slight air movement, i.e. normal indoor conditions. Clothing can be made with an insulating value of at least 6 Clo, although the provision of adequate insulation for the extremities in very cold conditions is always a problem.

The body's temperature sensors

The body has two distinct sets of temperature sensors: those which assess its core temperature and are thought to be located in the (probably anterior) hypothalamus; and those which sense its environmental temperature and are located in the skin. These two sets of sensors usually act together to maintain the body in thermal balance, but may at times produce conflicting signals, as when cold stimulation of the skin causes peripheral vasoconstriction and shivering even when the body's deep temperature is above normal. Many ingenious experiments have been performed to present conflicting stimuli to the central and peripheral temperature sensors; such experiments have increased considerably our knowledge of human temperature regulation, although many details have still to be elucidated.

Cutaneous receptors

Stimulation of the cutaneous temperature receptors may reach consciousness, and may thus produce a behavioural response, for example the changes of physical activity and social behaviour which play such an important part in human temperature regulation. In addition, stimulation of these receptors may initiate various subconscious reflex responses such as shivering, and changes in efferent sympathetic activity to the skin. It appears that stimulation of the cutaneous cold receptors causes reflex vasoconstriction and shivering; whereas stimulation of the hot receptors may (but not necessarily) cause reflex vasodilation.

Central receptors

Changes in deep-body temperature cause changes in the activity of various hypothalamic neurones. There appear to be two types of temperature-sensitive neurone in this area: one increases its firing rate in response to an *increase* of temperature, the other in response to a *decrease* of temperature. And stimulation of these neurones by changes in blood temperature causes reflex changes in the body's temperature—regulating mechanisms (see below).

There is at present much interest in the synaptic transmitters which are involved in the various neural interconnections of the hypothalamic temperature-regulating centres. This interest stems from experimental work in which injection of chemicals into the lateral ventricles of experimental animals has been shown to cause marked changes in thermal balance. This subject is however confused because substances which cause an increase of body temperature in one species cause a fall of temperature in another; and we have, of course, little understanding of the relevance of this work to temperature regulation in intact man. Possible hypothalamic transmitters include: adrenaline, noradrenaline and 5-hydroxytryptamine.

Thermoregulatory responses

The hypothalamus 'integrates' information about the body's core temperature (derived from its own temperature-sensitive neurones) with information from the cutaneous temperature receptors, and then initiates appropriate responses to maintain a constant deep-body temperature. In addition, in man, the cerebral cortex plays an important role in temperature regulation by bringing about appropriate behavioural responses, such as changes in the amount and type of clothing worn, or changes in physical activity. If there is clouding of consciousness for any reason these responses may not occur; and the person is then in danger of developing hypothermia when exposed to a cold environment (see later).

Response to cold environment

A decrease of body temperature causes reflex vasoconstriction in the peripheral parts of the body and therefore increases the effectiveness of its insulating shell. This response is mediated by sympathetically-induced vasoconstriction (see p. 16)

In a very cold environment, particularly during immersion in cold water, the body's vasoconstrictor response may be modified by the phenomenon of *cold vasodilatation*, in which the previously-constricted cutaneous vessels become widely dilated, thus increasing heat loss from the body. This vasodilatation is thought to result from a direct paralysing effect of cold on the restricted vessels; and it tends to be oscillatory, with the vessels alternately constricting and dilating. The advantage of this response to the body is dubious: by increasing the blood supply to the previously ischaemic tissues it may prevent tissue damge; but at the same time it reduces the amount of thermal insulation between the body's core and its environment, so that the danger of local gangrene is replaced by the danger of death from generalized hypothermia.

A fall in deep-body temperature of more than a degree or so causes an involuntary increase in heat production by shivering. This response may be induced also by intense stimulation of the cutaneous cold receptors, even when the core temperature is normal or above normal. As is the case with all muscular activity, the shivering response is mediated by nervous activity in the alpha motor neurones of the spinal cord; but the activity is thought to be transmitted down the cord not via the pyramidal tracts, but via the extra-pyramidal system, i.e. the reticulospinal and rubrospinal tracts.

Shivering can increase body metabolism by up to five times; this increase may however be insufficient to maintain thermal balance in a very cold environment. Also, shivering tends to be a relatively inefficient way of maintaining body temperature because the muscular activity increases blood flow to the limbs (and therefore increases peripheral heat loss), and the violent muscular movement disturbs the layer of relatively still air which surrounds the body and which normally provides much of its thermal insulation (see p. 171). In any case the active muscles tend to become fatigued; and the shivering mechanism fails when the deep-body temperature has reached about 33°C, being replaced by generalized muscular rigidity.

Response to warm environment

The body's response to a warm environment with an increase of body temperature is again partly behavioural and partly automatic. In a hot environment the prudent individual tends to wear light, loose clothing to aid convective heat loss and to minimize radiant heat gain, to minimize physical activity particularly in the heat of the day, and to take frequent cooling drinks.

The autonomic response to an increase of deep-body temperature takes the form of cutaneous vasodilatation, particularly of the arterio-venous anastomoses which link the arterioles and venules in the peripheral parts of the body. And this peripheral vasodilatation reduces the thermal insulating value of the body's superficial tissues, and so causes increased heat transfer between its central core and the colder environment.

If the body's core temperature rises appreciably, heat loss is increased by the onset of sweating; and, provided the environmental humidity is not too high, this mechanism permits the rapid loss of large amounts of heat. Sweating is controlled by the sympathetic nervous system: the peripheral transmitter is not however noradrenaline, as elsewhere in this system, but acetylcholine; and sweat production is consequently reduced by administration of atropine and similar drugs.

The latent heat evaporation of 1 g of water is about 2.4 kJ (0.6 Cal). To dissipate the body's normal heat production solely by evaporation of sweat (as is of course necessary when the environmental temperature exceeds 37°C—see p. 155), therefore requires the production of about 5 l sweat/24 hours. And when the body is gaining heat from thermal radiation and at the same time performing hard physical work the maintenance of thermal balance may require the production of as much as 10 l of sweat/24 hours.

To some extent, the ability to sweat profusely increases during prolonged exposure to a hot environment. This process is called heat acclimatization, another feature of which is reduction of the salt content of the sweat (see below). The concentration of sodium chloride in the sweat varies with the rate of sweat production, sodium intake, and the subject's heat acclimatization. It is affected also by the level of circulating aldosterone. Heat acclimatization results in a decreased sodium concentration in the sweat, and thus helps to conserve salt; but even so daily salt loss in a hot climate may amount to as much as 30 g (500 m mol).

Profuse sweating thus causes a severe loss from the body of both salt and water; and the resulting depletion of extracellular fluid volume may be sufficient to cause peripheral circulatory failure (see Chapter 2). Further, if the fluid lost is replaced simply by water this may result in haemodilution with symptoms of hyponatraemia (see Chapter 12) including painful muscle cramps ('stokers' cramps'). Fluid lost by sweating should be replaced by both salt and water; additional salt being conveniently administered in the form of salt tablets.

HYPOTHERMIA

When the body's physiological responses to cold are insufficient to maintain thermal balance body temperature falls, that is the patient develops hypothermia. Such a fall of deep-body temperature is of course particularly likely to occur in adverse environments, such as immersion in cold water, or exposure to wet-cold, for example during hill-walking in winter or deep sea diving. But hypothermia may occur also when the thermal stress is relatively mild, for example: in babies, who have a large body surface in relation to their metabolic mass and whose temperature-regulating mechanisms are poorly developed; during general anaesthesia, when the body's regulatory responses may be inactivated by drugs; in the elderly; and in patients with hypothyroidism (q.v.).

It is now well-recognized that minor degrees of hypothermia are relatively common in elderly patients who are living in poor socio-economic conditions; and it may well be that hypothermia is an important (but largely unrecognized) cause of death in the elderly. The reasons for the increased likelihood of elderly patients developing hypothermia is uncertain, but may include: depressed metabolism from sub-clinical degrees of hypothyroidism, impaired behavioural responses to cold, impaired autonomic responses to cold, and lack of money to provide adequate heating.

Clinical manifestations

The clinical manifestations of hypothermia are best seen in acute accidental hypothermia, for example following immersion in very cold water while wearing inadequate protective clothing*. The intense shivering which occurs initially is unable to increase bodily metabolism sufficiently to maintain thermal balance; and, depending on the clothing, body temperature falls more or less rapidly. As the deep-body temperature drops below about 33 °C there is increasing impairment of consciousness, leading ultimately to coma. The shivering response disappears and is replaced by generalized muscular rigidity, accompanied by a general depression of metabolism with reduction of body oxygen consumption, cardiac output and pulmon-

---

*Under these circumstances intense stimulation of cutaneous cold receptors causes a marked (reflex) increase in pulmonary ventilation; the victim is therefore totally unable to control his breathing, and is consequently in grave danger of drowning even before he has time to develop hypothermia. Life jackets are essential whenever there is a possibility of sudden immersion in very cold water.

ary ventilation. As the deep-body temperature falls below 30°C there is an increased incidence of cardiac arrhythmias with an increasing likelihood of ventricular fibrillation. Death usually occurs when the core temperature falls to around 28°C, although cases of recovery from much lower temperatures are on record (often in association with an excessive alcohol intake in the pre-hypothermic period).

Treatment

As in all things prevention is better than cure; and the prevention of accidental hypothermia requires clothing which is adequate and appropriate for the thermal environment. The insulating value of clothing falls dramatically if it becomes wet (see p. 170); and in the wet-cold situation it is necessary to keep dry by means of an external waterproof layer. (Care must be taken also to see that the clothing does not become saturated with sweat from the inside.)

The problem of preventing hypothermia is seen at its most severe in North Sea diving. Not only is the water wet (!) and very cold, but the use of helium-oxygen breathing mixtures* considerably enhances respiratory heat loss. It is now normal practice to heat the diver artificially by a heated diving suit, or by warm water piped from the surface.

There is some dispute about the best way to treat acute hypothermia, but most workers agree that the deep-body temperature should be raised as rapidly as possible by immersing the body in warm water (40 to 42°C naked, 44 to 46°C clothed). It is usually recommended that the limbs are kept out of the water lest cutaneous vasodilatation—by returning cold blood from the periphery to the central circulation—should cause a further drop of deep-body temperature ('after drop'). In exposed situations treatment along these lines is obviously difficult or impossible; and there is therefore much interest at present in the possibility of rewarming hypothermic patients by the inhalation of heated air or oxygen. One such system generates the necessary heat by the exothermic chemical reaction which occurs between carbon dioxide and soda lime.

There is less agreement about the best treatment for chronic hypothermia, but many workers suggest that the rewarming should take place slowly, for example by putting the patient into a warm bed and then letting his metabolic waste-heat do the rest. This treatment should be carried out only where there are adequate facilities for monitoring the patient's biochemistry and state of oxygenation.

---

*The thermal conductivity of helium is considerably greater than that of nitrogen.

HYPERTHERMIA (HYPERPYREXIA)

If the rate of heat loss from the body fails to keep pace with heat production (plus heat gain from the environment—see p. 000) body temperature must rise. This rise of temperature tends to produce a positive feedback situation (a 'vicious circle') because the increase of temperature increases body metabolism and thus heat production, and so tends to cause a further increase of body temperature. Failure of the sweating mechanism, as a result of dehydration for example, makes the situation worse, and results in a steep rise of body temperature and the condition of 'heat stroke' or hyperpyrexia.

Clinically, hyperpyrexia is characterized by a very high body temperature (41°C, or even higher), a hot dry skin, and evidence of central nervous system malfunction with disorientation, delirium, coma, muscle twitching, and even frank convulsions. The condition may be closely mimicked by *falciparum* malaria and other cerebral infections; and in endemic areas the former condition must always be excluded by examination of appropriate blood smears. Hyperpyrexia may occur also as a complication of cerebrovascular lesions particularly when these involve the pons; pontine haemorrhage being characterized by hyperpyrexia and bilateral pin-point pupils.

The loss of extracellular fluid which occurs with severe sweating tends to cause peripheral circulatory failure and a reduction of cardiac output (see Chapter 2). This, together with the fall of peripheral resistance which accompanies cutaneous vasodilatation, may produce a fall in arterial blood pressure sufficient to cause fainting—'heat syncope'.

Hyperpyrexia is particularly likely to occur when unacclimatized subjects are required to carry out hard physical work in a hot environment, particularly when the humidity is high; under these circumstances the only route by which the body can lose heat is by evaporation (see p. 173), and with a high environmental humidity this cannot occur. The condition can be precipitated also by lack of air movement, which impedes evaporation of sweat.

In addition to the circumstances considered above, hyperthermia occurs also as a *very rare* complication of general anaesthesia when an abnormality of muscle metabolism results, in the presence of certain anaesthetic agents, in a very considerable increase of heat production and a dramatic rise of deep-body temperature. This very serious, and often fatal, condition is known as 'malignant hyperpyrexia'.

Treatment

The treatment of hyperthermia is to cool the patient artificially as quickly as possible, otherwise the condition is likely to be rapidly fatal. Rapid cooling is achieved most easily by spraying the naked patient with cold water, and encouraging evaporation by fans. If the deep-body temperature is reduced to around 39°C—and assuming the condition is primary hyperthermia, and not merely a symptom of some other condition (see above)—the patient's own homeostatic mechanisms can then usually complete the process.

FEVER (PYREXIA)

Fever has been recognized as a clinical sign of disease—both infective and non-infective—for centuries. It now seems that the essential cause of this abnormality is that for some reason the body's 'thermostat' i.e. its hypothalamic temperature-regulating centre(s) have become 'reset' at a higher than normal temperature. This occurs typically as a result of the presence in the blood of fever-producing substances (pyrogens), which come either from the infecting organism itself, or from dead leucocytes and other phagocytes. Leucocyte pyrogen is thought to be a polypeptide with a molecular weight of between ten and twenty thousand.

Salicylates are thought to reduce or abolish the patient's fever by restoring the set-point of his hypothalamic temperature-regulating centre to normal. In recent years it has been found that injection of prostaglandin into the vicinity of an animal's hypothalamus causes fever which is *not* abolished by salicylates; and this has given rise to the hypothesis that pyrogens stimulate prostaglandin synthesis, and that a prostaglandin (probably prostaglandin E_2) is the ultimate cause of clinical pyrexia. Salicylates are thought to act by preventing the formation of this prostaglandin.

FURTHER READING

Anon. 1968 Heatstroke. British Medical Journal 2: 190

Anon. 1973 Extremes in heat or cold. Lancet 1: 1229

Anon. 1978 Rewarming for accidental hypothermia. Lancet i: 251

Collins K J 1977 Heat illness—diagnosis, treatment and prevention. Practitioner 219: 193

Cooper K E 1969 Regulation of body temperature. British Journal of Hospital Medicine 2: 1064

Cooper K E 1969 Fever. British Journal of Hospital Medicine 2: 1069

Coper K E 1972 Central mechanisms for the control of body temperature in health and febrile states. In: Modern trends in physiology 1. Butterworths, London

Cranston W I 1973 Fever. In: The scientific basis of medicine annual reviews. British Postgraduate Medical Federation

Dalgliesh D G 1972 Cold/wet exposure ashore. Journal of the Royal Naval Medical Service 58: 177

Exton-Smith A N 1973 Accidental hypothermia. British Medical Journal 4: 727

Fox R H 1974 Temperature regulation with special reference to man. In: Linden R J (Ed) Recent advances in physiology. Churchill Livingstone, Edinburgh and London, p 340

Fox R H, Woodward P M, Exton-Smith A N, Green M F, Donnison D V, Wicks M H 1941 A practical system of units for the determination of the heat exchange of man with his environment. Science 94: 428

Golden F St C 1972 Accidental hypothermia. Journal of the Royal Naval Medical Service 58: 196

Goldsmith R 1978 Acclimatisation to heat and cold in man. In: Baron D N, Compston N, Dawson A M (eds) Recent advances in medicine, 17th edn. Churchill Livingstone, Edinburgh and London

Hervey G R 1975 Physiological changes encountered in hypothermia. Proceedings of the Royal Society of Medicine 66: 1053

Hey E N 1972 Thermal regulation in the newborn. British Journal of Hospital Medicine 8: 51

Keatinge W R 1972 Cold immersion and swimming. Journal of the Royal Naval Medical Service 56: 171

Keatinge W R 1977 Accidental hypothermia and drowning. Practitioner 219: 183

Kew M C 1976 The effects of temperature change on the human body. British Journal of Hospital Medicine 16: 502

Lloyd E Ll 1973 Accidental hypothermia treated by central rewarming through the airway. British Journal of Anaesthesia 45: 41

Maclean D, Emslie-Smith D 1977 Accidental hypothermia. Blackwell, Oxford

Rawlin J S P 1972 Thermal balance in divers. Journal of the Royal Naval Medical Service 58: 182

14

Peripheral neurohumoral transmission and its disorders

The electrical and ionic changes accompanying propagation of the nerve impulse are now well established. The impulse, or action potential, is a travelling wave of electrical changes which results from movement of charged ions across the nerve membrane. The electrical changes consist of a loss, or 'depolarization' of the standing negative potential across the membrane which actually is 'reversed' and becomes positive for a fraction of a millisecond, followed by restoration of the negative potential, or 'repolarization'.

The chemical nature of the self-propagating change in structure of the nerve membrane underlying the action potential is not well understood. However, this change results in an alteration in the ionic permeability of the membrane, such that sodium ions can pass into the axon more easily, and it is this movement that initiates the action potential. Subsequently potassium and chloride ions can more easily pass outwards, and these movements are associated with restoration of the resting negative membrane potential.

It is generally held that similar changes accompany nerve activity in all nerve fibres both outside and within the central nervous system. In the case of myelinated fibres the process is modified since here the ionic permeability changes take place at the nodes of Ranvier only, and transmission between these nodes takes place by movement of ionic currents in a circuit including the core of the fibre and the surrounding extracellular fluid. This permits very much faster rates of conduction, e.g. up to 100 m/s, to be attained in these nerves. With the exception of the difference between myelinated and non-myelinated fibres the general principles of nerve conduction along an axon probably remain the same throughout the nervous system.

The situation is more complex in the case of transmission between, rather than within, neurones. There is now overwhelming evidence that transmission at nerve connections within the c.n.s (the so-called 'synapses'), at autonomic ganglia, at neuromuscular and other neuro-effector junctions, differs in many respects from the process of impulse propagation along the fibre. In all such junctions studied in vertebrates transmission involves the release of a chemical messenger, or 'neurohumour', which exerts an excitatory or inhibitory action on the next neurone in the chain. Since these interneuronal and neuro-effector junctions are the site of integration, by temporal and spatial summation, of activities in a number of incoming nerve pathways, it is perhaps to be expected that a specialized mechanism has evolved. What is perhaps more surprising, and at present unexplained, is why there should be a number of different mechanisms, using different neurohumours, at various sites in the peripheral and central nervous systems. This fact, however, has two important implications. Firstly, in at least one case in the peripheral nervous system (myasthenia gravis), in one case in the central nervous system (the Parkinsonian syndrome), and probably in further cases yet to be discovered, defects occur which appear to be relatively selective to one neurotransmitter mechanism. Secondly, that the action of a number of widely used drugs, particularly those acting on the autonomic nervous system, can be understood in terms of their interaction with specific mechanisms of neurohumoral transmission.

THE NEUROHUMORAL THEORY

Origination of the neurohumoral hypothesis is generally attributed to T. R. Elliott, who in 1905 drew attention to the similarities between the actions of the sympathetic division of the autonomic nervous system and the pharmacological effects of adrenaline. His hypothesis that the action of the sympathetic is mediated by an adrenaline-like substance released from nerve endings was doubted for many years, principally because it was regarded as unlikely that a mechanism involving the release, action and disposal of a chemical substance could act rapidly enough to effect the actions initiated by nerve activity. The principle of neurohumoral transmission is, however, now generally acknowledged, and certain experimental findings are accepted as necessary to demonstrate that a substance acts as a neurotransmitter in a particular site. These are:

1. The substance should be present within nerve endings.
2. Enzymatic mechanisms for synthesizing the substance should also be present within the nerve.
3. Activity of the nerve fibre should lead to release of the substance from nerve terminals.
4. Some mechanism for terminating the action of the substance should be present, e.g. enzymatic breakdown or specific uptake process.

5. Application of the substance to the postsynaptic or neuroeffector sites should mimic the effects of nerve activity.

These criteria are now well satisfied for acetylcholine at the neuro-muscular junction and some postganglionic parasympathetic neurones, and for noradrenaline at some, but not all, postganglionic sympathetic neurones. At those preganglionic sites which have been studied much evidence suggests that the transmitter substance here also is acetylcholine.

It has been widely held that either acetylcholine or noradrenaline acted as the chemical mediator of transmission at all junctions in the periphery. Recent evidence suggests, however, that particularly in the autonomic plexuses innervating the gut this may not be the case, and that other substances will have to be considered. For example peptides (e.g. vasoactive intestinal polypeptide, substance P and enkephalin) have been found in nerves and may have a neurotransmitter role. ATP, or a related substance, has also been suggested as a transmitter at some autonomic neuroeffector junctions.

Cholinergic and adrenergic transmission

Distribution

The sites at which acetylcholine and noradrenaline act as neurohu-mours are shown diagrammatically in Figure 25. The two divisions of the autonomic nervous system, the sympathetic and parasympathetic systems, each have two elements, a pre- and a postganglionic neurone, in their efferent connections. In either case, whether the ganglion is located proximally in the sympathetic chain and related ganglia, or distally in nerve networks in the viscus wall, as is usually the case with parasympathetic ganglia, the substance released by the preganglionic neurone is acetylcholine. This substance also is the postganglionic transmitter in the parasympathetic system in those sites which have at present been well studied. The neurohumour which fulfils this role for the sympathetic is, however, noradrenaline, the similarities between the pharmacological actions of this substance and adrenaline being sufficiently close to explain the essential correctness of Elliott's original hypothesis. There are nevertheless two well-established exceptions to this rule. The innervation of the sweat glands, and the vasodilator fibres to skeletal muscle, are both activated from the thoraco-lumbar, or sympathetic, portion of the autonomic system, yet both seem likely to release acetylcholine at the neuroeffector junction.

The medulla of the adrenal gland is morphologically equivalent to a postganglionic element of the sympathetic system, and its chromaffin

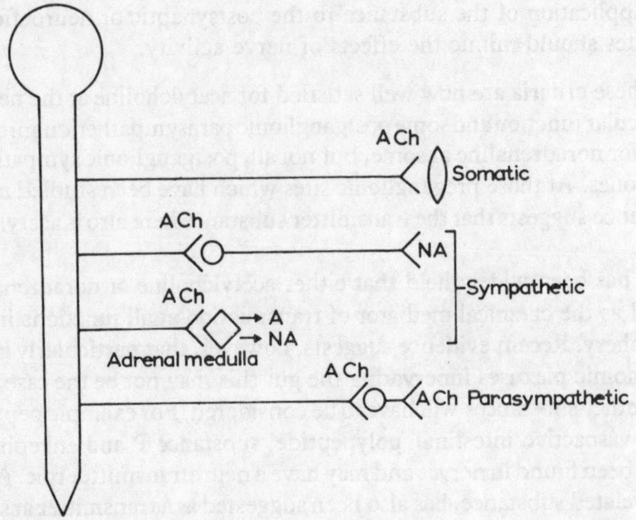

Fig. 25 Sites of release of acetylcholine (ACh), adrenaline (A), and noradrenaline (NA) in the peripheral nervous system.

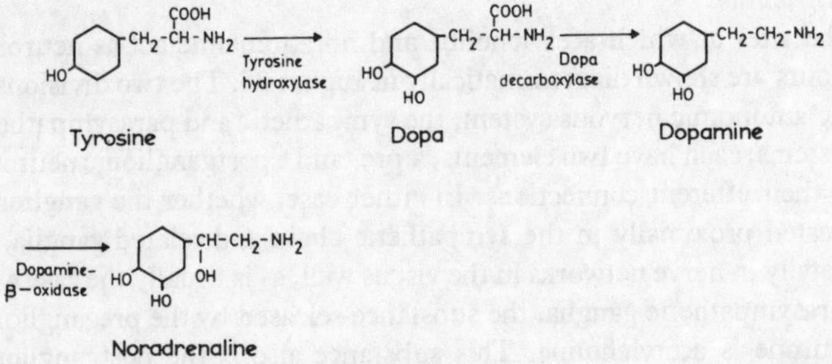

Fig. 26. Synthetic pathway for the catecholamines, dopamine and noradrenaline.

cells release a mixture of adrenaline and noradrenaline in response to activation of its cholinergic 'preganglionic' innervation.

Mechanism of release
The substances acetylcholine and noradrenaline are synthesized within the nerve endings from the respective precursor substances choline and tyrosine. In the former case this is accomplished by the enzyme choline acetyltransferase, and in the latter by the sequence of enzymatic reactions shown in Figure 26. The rates of synthesis are regulated by a feedback mechanism from nerve activity so that an increased rate of synthesis follows periods of rapid nerve firing. A

number of lines of evidence suggest that the two neurotransmitter substances themselves are stored in the nerve ending within subcellular particles. Such particles are visible with the electron microscope and are referred to as vesicles in cholinergic, and as granules in adrenergic, nerves.

The mechanism whereby nerve activity releases the neurotransmitter from its storage sites is ill-understood but has been most closely studied at the cholinergic neuromuscular junction. Here Katz and his colleagues have shown that the process requires the presence of calcium ions in the extracellular fluid. They have also shown that when the junction is viewed from a recording electrode situated within the muscle fibre close to the motor end-plate small excitations of miniature end-plate potentials (M.E.P.P.s), similar in form to, but of much smaller magnitude than, the end-plate potential (E.P.P.) which results from nerve activity, can be observed even when the nerve is completely inactive. These M.E.P.P.s probably represent the spontaneous release of small quanta, or 'packets', of acetylcholine, and it is thought that one quantum may correspond to the contents of one vesicle in the nerve teminal. The end-plate potential itself represents the very rapid release of a larger number of such quanta, and it is possible, but not proved, that the arrival of a nerve impulse at the nerve terminal somehow provokes the release into the junctional cleft of the contents of many acetylcholine-containing vesicles by a process of exocytosis.

Mechanism of disposal

There is evidence that the release of the two neurotransmitters is in many respects similar, but in the mechanisms of disposal there are certain important differences. It has long been recognized that the action of acetylcholine is terminated primarily by an enzyme, known as acetylcholinesterase, which acts by hydrolysing the active chemical molecule. Indeed, investigations of the mode of action of the drug physostigmine (Eserine), an inhibitor of acetylcholinesterase, were historically of crucial importance in establishing the neurohumoral theory. The enzyme itself has been shown to be located both at pre- and postjunctional sites at the neuromuscular junction, and particularly in the latter situation it is well placed to inactivate acetylcholine immediately after it has depolarized the motor end-plate. The action of the neurotransmitter in normal circumstances is thus limited in time, destruction taking place within milliseconds, and in place, to the region of the motor end-plate.

While it had been widely expected that similar mechanisms would be operative at the adrenergic neuroeffector junction, this is probably not the case. It is true that there are enzymic systems which metabolize noradrenaline released from nerve endings, catechol-o-methyltransferase being one such enzyme, but it appears that their action is neither as rapid as in the case of cholinesterase, nor as well localized to the postjunctional site. Indeed, pharmacological inhibition of these enzymes is without significant effect on adrenergic transmission, which is in striking contrast to the effects of inhibition of acetylcholinesterase on cholinergic transmission.

It is probable that the main disposal mechanism for noradrenaline is a specific uptake process which concentrates the neurotransmitter in noradrenergic nerve terminals and thereby removes it from the site of its action. The evidence for the existence of the uptake process is that all adrenergically innervated tissues have a large capacity to take up infused noradrenaline, and this capacity is much reduced after section and degeneration of the nerve supply. Various other experiments using histo-chemical and autoradiographic techniques also agree in finding that the adrenergic terminals possess a powerful mechanism for assimilating the amine against a concentration gradient. It is very likely, therefore, that this is the major method of disposal for noradrenaline released from terminals by nerve activity. The potential clinical significance of the mechanism lies in the fact that a number of drugs including the iminodibenzyl group of compounds (the tricyclic 'antidepressants'—see Chapter 15) are able to inhibit this uptake process, and this inhibition may be at the basis of some of their pharmacological actions. Recently it has been recognized that release of noradrenaline is regulated by receptors (the α_2 receptors) located on the presynaptic neurone. Thus drugs such as clonidine which stimulate noradrenergic receptors may inhibit noradrenaline release.

MYASTHENIA GRAVIS AS A DEFECT IN CHOLINERGIC TRANSMISSION

In 1934 Dr Mary Walker predicted that, because there are similarities between the actions of curare, which blocks the effects of acetylcholine at the neuromuscular junction, and the symptoms of myasthenia gravis, these symptoms might be improved by potentiation of cholinergic transmission by the administration of the acetylcholinesterase inhibitor physostigmine (Eserine). This proved to be correct, and subsequent therapeutic results in, and investigations of, this condition have supported the concept that there is a defect in cholinergic transmission at the neuromuscular junction.

The most characteristic clinical feature is abnormal fatigability and weakness of skeletal muscles increasing with usage and towards the end of the day. When recordings are made through electrodes within the muscles themselves, by the technique of electro-myography, there is a rapid decline in the amplitude of the potentials resulting from continued nerve stimulation. This finding indicates the failure of a fixed size of volley of nerve activity to continue to evoke activity in the same number of muscle fibres. The failure is restored, at least partially, by administration of the acetylcholinesterase inhibitor physostigmine which presumably has the effect of prolonging the action of acetylcholine at the motor end-plate.

One might postulate that the site of the effect was either prejunctional, e.g. insufficient quantities of acetylcholine are released by sustained nerve activity, or postjunctional, e.g. that some curare-like substance blocked the motor end-plate and that this blockade could only be overcome by increased amounts of acetylcholine, such as might be achieved in the presence of an anticholinesterase agent. If the defect were of the latter type, i.e. that the end-plates were abnormally insensitive, then it is difficult to see why the characteristic fatigue effect occurs. However, there is evidence that patients with myasthenia are abnormally insensitive to intra-arterial injections of acetylcholine. If the defect were at the presynaptic site it seems possible that it might be of such a nature that whereas the first action potentials in a chain of nerve impulses are able to mobilize enough acetylcholine, the mechanism becomes exhausted by repetitive activity. Direct investigation in humans is difficult, but there is some evidence for defective release of acetylcholine in biopsy specimens taken from myasthenic subjects. It has been claimed both that the quantity of acetylcholine released is low and also that the size of the M.E.P.P.s recorded from such specimens, but not their number, is reduced.

The cause, or underlying pathogenesis, of the defective transmission has also been the centre of debate. The generalized nature of the disease suggests the presence of some circulating toxic humoral factor, and consistent with this possibility is the fact that a transient 'neonatal' form of the disease is sometimes seen in the first few days of life in infants born to myasthenic mothers. Recently it has been found that at least 70 per cent of patients with myasthenia have antibodies directed at this acetylcholine receptor itself. Moreover, animals immunised with acetylcholine may develop a syndrome resembling myasthenia, and serum from such animals has neuromuscular blocking activity. These findings rather strongly support the view that the defect is at the acetylcholine receptor.

Treatment of myasthenia

The drug treatment of myasthenia was revolutionized by Mary Walker's discovery, and the principle of the use of anticholinesterases remains the same. Sufficient quantities of anticholinesterase are administered to increase the effectiveness of nerve activity to the optimal level which can be achieved without the appearance of incapacitating side effects. The anticholinesterases themselves can be divided into two groups: the reversible inhibitors, such as physostigmine, neostigmine, and pyridostigmine—a group which includes all those drugs used therapeutically—and the non-reversible compounds such as Dyflos and other organophosphorus compounds, some of which have a use as insecticides. The mode of action of the former is by competitive inhibition, the compounds themselves resembling acetylcholine in structure and acting as substrates for cholinesterase, whilst the latter form a stable compound with, and thus inactivate, the enzyme.

The side effects of anticholinesterase therapy fall into two groups and can be predicted on physiological gounds. The *first group* arises from the fact that the drug action cannot be limited to the neuromuscular junction but must also influence autonomic sites, and particularly the parasympathetic neuroeffector junctions. Pupilloconstriction, increased exocrine secretion, bradycardia, bronchoconstriction, and increased gut movements thus are common manifestations, and may be indicators of too large a dose. These actions may be regarded as an inevitable consequence of the fact that actylcholine has a function elsewhere than at the neuromuscular junction; (it is interesting to note in passing that as far as is known the myasthenic process does not affect autonomic cholinergic mechanisms). The *second group* of side effects arises from the fact that excessive activity at the neuromuscular junction can have the reverse of the desired effect if acetylcholine persists to the extent of producing the so-called 'depolarization block'. In this case the persistent presence of acetylcholine results in continued depolarization of the motor end-plate, and failure of muscle contraction. This causes increasing muscular weakness. The clinical problem may be therefore to distinguish increased weakness resulting from the disease ('myasthenic crisis') from that due to treatment. The short-acting anticholinesterase edrophonium (Tensilon) is sometimes administered in this situation, an improvement in muscle power indicating a myasthenic crisis rather than an anticholinesterase excess. This procedure has the substantial disadvantage that in the case of a drug-induced weakness the situation will be made worse, and facilities for dealing with this eventuality (e.g. assisted respiration) must be available (see section on respiratory failure.)

OTHER POSSIBLE DEFECTS OF TRANSMISSION

Myasthenia is a relatively uncommon disease. Two other defects, while much rarer, are also of interest in that they seem to involve relatively selective disorders of peripheral autonomic function, and may possibly be associated with defects of neurohumoral transmission, although the nature and site of such defects have yet to be elucidated.

The first of these, familial dysautonomia (the Riley-Day syndrome), is inherited as a recessive condition, and has been described predominantly in children of the Jewish race. Many features of this condition relate to the autonomic system and include some features, such as defective tear-secretion and postural hypotension, suggestive of hypofunction, and others, like hyperhidrosis and increased gastrointestinal motility, which suggest hyperfunction. These various features are difficult to explain simply in terms of present concepts of autonomic function. However, the possibility that a neurohumoral defect may be present is raised by the finding of a decrease in the excretion of the noradrenaline metabolite vanillyl-mandelic acid, and an increase in the excretion of homovanillic acid, the metabolite of the precursor dopamine. A defect of conversion of dopamine to noradrenaline is therefore a possiblity but would not explain all the clinical features.

In the second syndrome, primary autonomic degeneration (the Shy-Drager syndrome), features of autonomic disorder may be combined with basal ganglia dysfunction. In some cases the defect appears to lie in the peripheral adrenergic neurone, and circulating levels of noradrenaline are low. In other cases the defect in autonomic control is at a higher level. Severe postural hypotension and defective sweating in these cases seems to be attributable to degeneration of cells of the intermediolateral column of the spinal cord, i.e. of the cell bodies of the preganglionic elements of the sympathetic nervous system. There is also defective sphincter control, which probably reflects a disorder of parasympathetic function. That these defects should be combined with central nervous dysfunctions, frequently with the Parkinsonian syndrome, is of great interest in view of the evidence for specific neurochemical disturbances in the latter disorder (see Chapter 15). There must presumably be some common structural factor in the systems involved, but what this may be is at present unknown.

Neither of these disorders of the autonomic system is as well understood as myasthenia, nor as accessible to drug therapy. Their features suggest, however, that other specific disorders of peripheral neural transmission exist and may be clarified by further understanding of autonomic control.

FURTHER READING

Axelrod J 1971 Noradrenaline: fate and control of its biosynthesis. Science, New York 173: 598

Bannister R R 1979 Chronic autonomic failure with postural hypotension. Lancet ii: 404

Desmedt J E 1966 Presynaptic mechanisms in myasthenia gravis. Annals of the New York Academy of Sciences 135: 209

Euler U S von 1971 Adrenergic neurotransmitter functions. Science, New York 173: 202

Grob D 1976 Cause of weakness in myasthenia gravis. New England Journal of Medicine 294: 722

Havard C W H 1977 Progress in myasthenia gravis. British Medical Journal ii: 1008

Katz B 1971 Quantal mechanism of neural transmitter release. Science, New York 173: 123

Ziegler M G, Lake C R, Kopin I J 1977 The sympathetic-nervous-system defect in primary orthostatic hypotension. New England Journal of Medicine 296: 293

15

Disorders of aminergic transmission in the central nervous system

The contribution of physiology to understanding disease processes is perhaps least in the case of the central nervous system. Whereas thorough neuroanatomical knowledge is necessary to understand the effects of localized lesions, quite crude concepts of nerve function are probably as useful in understanding neurological disease as a detailed acquaintance with much modern neurophysiological research. The reasons for this no doubt include the complexity of the nervous system and the obscure nature of many of the diseases which afflict it, but for these same reasons the interaction between advancing knowledge of clinical disorders and basic research when it occurs is perhaps more immediate and has a greater impact than in other fields. One area where such interactions currently are taking place is in the field of neuropharmacology where there have been a number of recent advances relevant to understanding c.n.s. diseases and their treatment.

Since the development of the neurohumoral theory of peripheral transmission (see Chapter 14) it has been widely suspected that similar principles of chemical transmission must also apply within the central nervous system. In the past ten years evidence has accumulated that at least seven different substances—acetylcholine, noradrenaline, adrenaline, dopamine, 5-hydroxytryptamine, γ-aminobutyric acid and glycine—can be said to be very likely to have a neurotransmitter role in the c.n.s. according to the criteria enumerated in Chapter 14 (p. 184) There is also now a strong case that a number of peptides (e.g., enkephalin, substance P) act as neurotransmitters in the same or a similar way to the smaller molecular weight substances already established as neurohumours. For other substances (e.g. glutamic acid) the evidence is suggestive. The emerging pattern is certainly complex and provokes the questions of what functional significance there may be in the pattern of distribution of transmitters in the brain, and whether it is possible that certain central nervous diseases, whose etiology is at present obscure, may be associated with specific neurotransmitter dysfunctions comparable to the myasthenic defect in the peripheral nervous system. The existence of a number of distinct neurohumoral systems suggests that it may be possible to manipulate these mechanisms by specific chemical means, and that a rational science of neuropharmacology can be hoped for.

In Parkinson's disease clinical progress has recently been paralleled by basic research to the extent that explanations of important advances in drug therapy can now be framed in anatomical and biochemical terms. This is very largely due to progress in understanding monoaminergic mechanisms in the brain. Whereas a major problem in neurotransmitter research is to determine the precise anatomical pathways from which particular transmitters are released, this question has been largely solved for the substances noradrenaline, dopamine, and 5-hydroxytryptamine by the development of a specific histochemical technique. The main anatomical features of the monoamine-containing pathways in the brain have been described and their physiology to a certain extent illuminated.

STRUCTURE AND FUNCTION OF MONOAMINE-CONTAINING NEURONES

Anatomy

With tissue prepared according to the Falck-Hillarp histochemical technique it is possible to demonstrate specific fluorescence in those areas of the brain where one of the monoamines, noradrenaline, dopamine or 5-hydroxytryptamine, is located. Such studies show these substances to be present within three specific sets of neurones and that each set of neurones has high concentrations of the particular amine within the diffusely distributed terminal systems and moderate concentrations within the cell bodies. The principal findings of such studies are illustrated diagrammatically in Figure 27.

They may be summarized as follows:
1. Several discrete groups of cell bodies are located at various sites within the brainstem.
2. Noradrenaline- and 5-hydroxytryptamine-containing cell bodies, mainly in the caudal brainstem, give rise to descending fibre systems with a terminal distribution within the grey matter of the spinal cord.
3. Noradrenaline- and 5-hydroxytryptamine-containing cell bodies, mainly in the rostral brainstem, give rise to ascending fibre systems which travel through the lateral hypothalamus to terminal systems with a widespread distribution which includes various hypothalamic nuclei and the neocortex.
4. Dopamine-containing cell bodies are located mainly in a large group which encompasses the pars compacta of the substantia nigra

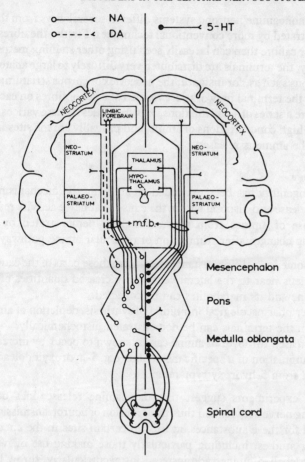

Fig. 27. Major monoamine-containing pathways in the c.n.s., according to Anden *et al.* (1966), Acta physiologica scandinavia 67, 313, DA, dopamine; NA, noradrenaline; 5-HT, 5-hydroxytryptamine; m.f.b., medial forebrain bundle.

and the region over the interpeduncluar nucleus in the ventral mesencephalon. They give rise to fibre systems which travel through the lateral hypothalamus to be distributed to terminals in the corpus striatum and some related nuclei in the septal region ('limbic forebrain'), and some areas of frontal cortex.

Recent work making use of immunohistochemical methods for localizing the enzyme phenylethanolamine-N-methyl transferase, which converts noradrenaline to adrenaline, suggests that some amine-containing neurones arising from cell bodies in the caudal brainstem and giving rise to terminals in hypothalamic areas probably release adrenaline, rather than noradrenaline, as a neurotransmitter.

The monoamine neurone systems differ in several ways from those demonstrated by more conventional techniques. Firstly, the fibres are of a finer calibre than can be easily seen using other staining methods; secondly, the terminals are distributed very diffusely to large anatomical regions such as, for instance, the neocortex or corpus striatum; and thirdly, the terminal networks are formed of a net of fibres on each of which are a series of small dilations, or 'varicosities'. These varicosities contain high concentrations of amine, and probably are the sites from which the amine is released.

Physiology

Much ingenuity has been expended on studying the mechanisms of amine release and disposal within the c.n.s. That nerve activity results in release of amines from the terminals is demonstrated by the following changes after stimulation of particular amine pathways:

(a) In some special circumstances (e.g. from those parts of the caudate nucleus near to the lateral ventricle) increased quantities of the amine and its metabolites can be collected.

(b) After pharmacological inhibition of synthesis, depletion of amine from the terminals can be demonstrated histochemically.

(c) Increased turnover of amine can be shown to occur by increased accumulation of a specific metabolite (e.g. 5-hydroxyindoleacetic acid from 5-hydroxytryptamine).

Such experiments suggest that monoamine release does occur following nerve activity and thus this criterion of neurotransmission is fulfilled for these substances, at least in certain sites in the c.n.s.

Other studies, including particularly those making use of radioactively labelled amines adminstered intraventricularly, throw light on the probable mechanisms of disposal. These studies show that each set of neurones containing a particular amine has a specific affinity or uptake process similar to that which has been demonstrated for noradrenaline in the peripheral sympathetic postganglionic neurone. The process in each case is specific, but only relatively so, for the particular amine synthesized in the neurone; and the possible significance of this specificity is that the uptake mechanisms can be inhibited by various pharmacological agents. If, as seems likely, the uptake process is the major mechanism for removing transmitter released as a result of nerve activity then, it has been argued, blockade of the uptake process may increase the concentration of the transmitter at its active site and thus potentiate the effects of nerve activity.

A major unsolved problem concerns the normal functional role of the amine systems. Despite a fairly large amount of experimentation in recent years no overall pattern has yet emerged although certain experimental findings in lesioning and stimulation studies are suggestive. Some major findings at the present time are that:

(i) decreases of 5-hydroxytryptamine in the forebrain, whether brought about by lesions of the ascending 5-hydroxytryptamine-containing neurones or by pharmacological means are accompanied by a decrease in total sleep-time. On this basis it has been suggested that the 5-hydroxytryptamine-containing neurones are concerned in regulating, or perhaps initiating, sleep;

(ii) lesions, including relatively specific lesions of catecholamine-containing neurones produced by the chemical 6-hydroxy-dopamine, that interrupt the dopamine-containing neurones ascending to the corpus striatum have the effect of producing marked akinesia, and also interfere with food and water intake;

(iii) stimulation through electrodes placed amongst the dopamine-containing fibres or cell bodies results in an increase in motor activity. Rats with electrodes in these sites can also be trained to press a lever to deliver trains of stimuli through their own implanted electrodes (the 'self-stimulation' phenomenon), and therefore this behaviour may also depend on activation of dopamine-containing neurones. These observations suggest that the dopamine-containing neurones may function as a 'motor-activating system', and may also possibly be concerned with mediating the effects of rewarding stimuli on behaviour;

(iv) similar studies with electrodes implanted in relation to one set of noradrenaline-containing neurones (those arising from the locus coeruleus in the mid pons) suggest that activation of these neurones may also support 'self-stimulation' behaviour, although in this case there are no striking increases in motor activity following stimulation. There may therefore be two sets of catecholamine-containing neurones (one dopamine—and one noradrenaline-containing) which act as neural 'reward' systems.

Such experiments do no more than provide a suggestion of the functional significance of the amine neurones. It would appear, however, that their functions are of a very general and fundamental nature, and it might therefore be predicted that disturbances in their function, whether induced by a disease process or by drug administration, would result in widespread changes in total activity and other aspects of behaviour.

PARKINSON'S DISEASE

Pathophysiology of Parkinson's disease

A striking, and not uncommon, clinical picture encountered in neurology is that of paralysis agitans, a syndrome first clearly delineated by James Parkinson in 1817. The cardinal features of this disorder are a triad of rigidity, tremor, and hypo- (or brady-) kinesia, or slowness of movement. They thus lie in the field of motor control. But it has long been recognized that they cannot be attributed to any simple dysfunction of the classical descending motor pathway, the pyramidal tracts. Therefore the disease has been regarded as one which affects the vaguely defined and ill-understood 'extrapyramidal' motor system, although the site of the lesions and the mode of production of symptoms has until recently remained obscure.

Important light has been shed on these questions by biochemical studies. That the core of the disease might lie in a chemical dysfunction was foreshadowed by the fact that a syndrome, in many respects identical to that occurring idiopathically, has frequently been observed following administration of certain psychotropic drugs. The phenothiazine and butyrophenone drugs in large doses can all provoke a classical Parkinsonian syndrome, and this picture has also been observed following administration of the hypotensive agents reserpine, tetrabenazine and α-methyl-dopa, all of which have actions on central amine-containing neurones.

The possibility that a defect in monoaminergic transmission might underlie one of the 'extrapyramidal' syndromes was opened up by the discovery that the substance dopamine was concentrated mainly within the major structure of the basal ganglia, the corpus striatum (comprising the caudate nucleus and the putamen, which are separated by the internal capsule). Ehringer and Hornykiewicz in 1960 made the important finding that in the brains of patients who had died from Parkinson's disease the concentration of dopamine in the corpus striatum was markedly lower than in the brains of control subjects dying from other causes. The concentrations of noradrenaline and 5-hydroxytryptamine were also reduced but to a much lesser degree, and in subsequent investigations it was demonstrated that the levels of these amines, but not that of dopamine, could be returned to normal values or above by treatment with monoamine oxidase inhibiting drugs. From these investigations it appeared that some, or perhaps all, cases of the syndrome of Parkinsonism might be associated with a specific depletion of the amine dopamine in that site in the corpus striatum where it is known from histochemical studies that it is concentrated within the varicosities of the terminals of nerve fibres originating in cell bodies in the ventral mesencephalon.

The cause of the striking depletion of dopamine in the corpus striatum remains obscure, but it is clearly a possibility that some degenerative process has had a selective effect on the dopamine neurones. In support of this theory there is neuropathological evidence, much of it dating from the period before the description of the amine-containing neurones, to suggest that in some cases of Parkinson's disease there is a loss of cells in the substantia nigra, the region of the dopamine-containing cell bodies.

The 'dopamine-deficiency' hypothesis of Parkinsonism is therefore the view that the characteristic defects in this syndrome arise from a deficiency of functional dopamine at synapses in the corpus striatum, although how the specific symptoms arise, or whether all three components can be attributed to one particular deficiency, is not entirely clear. Consistent with the hypothesis, however, is the occasional occurrence of a Parkinsonian syndrome following reserpine or tetrabenazine treatment, both of which drugs may cause a decrease in striatal dopamine levels, in addition to decreases in the other two amines elsewhere in the brain. An iatrogenic Parkinsonian syndrome is, in fact, much more commonly caused by the phenothiazines, but these drugs have no depleting effect on cerebral dopamine stores, although they probably increase the rate at which a major metabolite of this amine—homovanillic acid—accumulates. The explanation currently favoured is that the phenothiazines interfere with dopaminergic transmission, not by depleting presynaptic amine stores, as do reserpine and tetrabenazine, but by blocking the postsynaptic site in the corpus striatum, in a manner somewhat similar to that in which curare blocks the effect of acetylcholine at the neuromuscular junction. Blockade of dopamine receptors appear to elicit a feedback process which activates the pre-synaptic dopamine neurone and thus increases dopamine release and metabolism.

Evidence for this view that neuroleptics block dopamine receptors comes from experiments on the interactions of drugs with aminergic mechanisms in animals. The amphetamines and related drugs release dopamine from striatal nerve terminals and produce characteristic behavioural changes. These are effectively blocked by the phenothiazines, as also are the very similar behavioural changes elicited by apomorphine administration. The apomorphine effects are not inhibited by drug-induced inhibition of amine synthesis, and this suggests that apomorphine may act as a direct 'dopamine receptor stimulator'. That the major effects of both apomorphine and the amphetamines are blocked by phenothiazine administration is therefore consistent with the view that the phenothiazine drugs are able to induce dopamine receptor blockade.

Pharmacotherapy of the Parkinsonian syndrome

A direct confirmation of the 'dopamine deficiency' hypothesis of the Parkinsonian defect would be the demonstration that restoration of dopaminergic function to normal levels has the effect of reversing the clinical symptoms. Measurement of biochemical changes taking place in the striatum in human subjects in life is not yet feasible, but the possibility of influencing dopaminergic transmission in a therapeutic manner led first Hornykiewicz, and later other workers, to assess the effects of administration of L-DOPA, the catecholamine precursor. Administration of dopamine itself, as of the other cerebral monoamines, is without significant effect on the central nervous system as in normal circumstances an effective 'blood-brain barrier', probably located mainly in the capillary pericytes, prevents these substances from gaining access to the brain (Fig. 28). The precursor L-DOPA, however, is not limited in this way and it seemed possible, although perhaps *a priori* unlikely if the basic damage to the nervous system involves degeneration of amine-containing neurones, that administration of L-DOPA might increase dopamine turnover and thus restore towards normal the defectively functioning system. Early results were unimpressive, but in 1967 Cotzias and his colleagues proposed the introduction of much higher doses than had previously been used. Since this date it has become increasingly clear that the use of L-DOPA produces changes in some cases of Parkinson's disease superior to those brought about by other drugs or by surgical means, and L-DOPA now occupies a major and central role in therapy, and in particular is able in some cases to reverse the bradykinesia, which has been refractory to other methods of treatment.

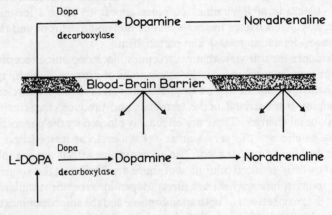

Fig. 28. Passage of L-DOPA into brian tissue (after F. K. Goodwin, 1971, Seminars in Psychiatry, 3, 477.)

Although the 'dopamine deficiency' hypothesis was the rationale for introducing L-DOPA, it does not necessarily follow that the therapeutic benefits result from an increase of cerebral dopamine. Indeed, if the dopamine-containing neurones have degenerated, the capacity for converting L-DOPA into dopamine, which depends on the presence of the enzyme aromatic L-amino-decarboxylase, is probably diminished, since this enzyme is located within the amine-containing neurones. It is possible that enough neurones survive to decarboxylate sufficient of the precursor substance, or alternatively, it has been suggested, decarboxylation may take place elsewhere in the nervous system, e.g. in neighbouring cells or in the capillary endothelium, which possesses high concentrations of the decarboxylase. Either of these possibilities would be consistent with the theory that the therapeutic effects are mediated by dopamine formation. It cannot be excluded, however, at the present time, that some other mechanism such as increased sensitivity of the 'denervated' dopamine receptor to L-DOPA itself is involved.

The side effects of L-DOPA are not easy to explain in terms of present concepts. Among the central effects choreoathetosis and dyskinesias, particularly involving the oral and facial musculature, are well recognized signs of overdosage. The physiopathology of such disordered movements is obscure, but when occurring in other conditions they have sometimes been improved by administration of amine-depleting drugs. Nausea and vomiting are probably central in origin as they occur in subjects given intravenous infusions of L-DOPA, and it is of interest that apomorphine, mentioned above as a possible dopamine receptor stimulant, is also a powerful centrally-acting emetic agent. It is likely that a dopamine receptor is located in the vomiting centre in the caudal brainstem.

Peripheral autonomic side effects are also complex. It might be expected that the presence in excess of the precursor of noradrenaline would lead to increased sympathetic tone and thus, perhaps to a rise in blood pressure. Such effects do not occur, perhaps partly because transmitter release is dependent upon nerve activity, and largely independent of precursor availability. On the contrary, hypotensive effects of L-DOPA are common and troublesome. Several possible explanations have been proposed:

1. The dopamine-β-oxidase step in noradrenaline synthesis is overwhelmed, with the result that dopamine as well as noradrenaline accumulates in the transmitter storage packets in the nerve ending. Nerve activity in this case might release a mixture of both substances with less pressor effect than noradrenaline alone.

2. The fall in tissue noradrenaline levels observed in studies of DOPA administration in animals occurs also in man, and as a result vasoconstrictor nerve activity may be less effective.

3. Dopamine is formed in excess in subjects treated with L-DOPA, and release of this substance into the circulation has a hypotensive action. It is known from animal experiments that intravenous injections of dopamine can have such an effect, and this action is blocked by phenothiazines.

It has also been shown that in some Parkinsonian patients the renin-angiotensin mechanism for blood pressure control (see Chapter 3) is impaired, and this may make such patients more susceptible to alterations in noradrenaline synthesis and release.

L-DOPA has been widely used since 1968. Drugs with an anticholinergic atropine-like effect, including such compounds as orphenadrine, benzhexol, and benztropine, have a much longer history in the therapy of Parkinsonism and usually have some effect on the tremor and rigidity of the disease, although ineffective against akinesia. Their ability to block central cholinergic mechanisms is probably related to their efficacy since the symptoms of Parkinsonism are exacerbated by the anticholinesterase physostigmine, which enters the c.n.s., but are not affected by edrophonium, which does not. Moreover this exacerbation is antagonized by the atropine-like compound scopolamine, which reaches the brain, but not by methylscopolamine, which does not.

These findings suggest that central cholinergic mechanisms must also be involved in the phenomena of Parkinsonism, and it has been suggested that a dopamine-acetylcholine balance exists in the basal ganglia, and that the symptoms arise when cholinergic activity is in relative excess. In this case the balance could be restored either by increasing the dopaminergic elements, as by L-DOPA therapy, or by reducing the cholinergic effects as by administering drugs with an atropine-like action. However, the fact that the spectrum of activity of the two therapies is somewhat different argues against any very simple interpretation of their modes of action. Information on central cholinergic mechanisms is in some respects not so far advanced as that concerning monoaminergic transmission. Both acetylcholine and choline acetylase are present in high concentration in the basal ganglia, but techniques for determining precisely which pathways in the c.n.s. utilize acetylcholine as a transmitter have not yet been developed.

AMINERGIC MECHANISMS AND PSYCHIATRIC DISORDER

The success of recent experiments in elucidating the mechanisms of neurohumoral transmission and particularly in relating the Parkinsonian syndrome to defective dopaminergic mechanisms in the basal ganglia, provokes the question of whether there exist other relatively specific neurotransmitter defects which may lie at the basis of some as yet obscure diseases. Perhaps the main interest of this possibility is that, while it is difficult at the present time to see any serious prospect of repairing structural defects in the c.n.s., the possibility of ameliorating specific chemical disorders by pharmacological means seems more feasible.

The hypothesis of specific chemical defects has been energetically pursued in the field of psychiatric disorder. Indeed, historically much recent work on central aminergic mechanisms can be seen to have stemmed from the discovery, and investigation of the mode of action, of the drug reserpine; and the finding that it has both some therapeutic usefulness in psychiatry and some undesirable side effects in its actions on mental function. Studies on reserpine's amine-depleting actions have provoked a number of hypotheses about the nature of particular psychiatric disorders which are currently under investigation.

Amongst the psychoses—the more serious forms of psychiatric disorder—two major distortions of mental function are recognized, In the *affective disorders*, a category which includes the severer depressive illnesses, the core feature is held to be a disturbance of 'mood', although this commonly is associated with somatic symptoms such as disturbance of appetite, sleep, and menstruation. The mood change, when it is in a depressive direction, is manifested by an altered responsiveness to the environment such that the individual reacts to stimuli, which previously would have been rewarding, either with a lack of interest, or with hostility and aggression. In the *schizophrenias*, on the other hand, which many regard as probably of multiple etiology, the disturbance of mental function, while it may include disorders of mood, extends also into the fields of perception and cognition, so that hallucinations, a disorder of perception, and delusions, a distortion in the interpretation of sensory experience, commonly occur.

Neither the affective nor the schizophrenic types of disturbance are usually associated with focal neurological defects but they consist rather of a generalized disturbance of higher nervous function. The evidence that the monoamine-containing neurones subserve rather general behavioural functions and have a diffuse distribution within the prosencephalon therefore makes it plausible that defects of these pathways might be manifest in generalized psychiatric disturbance. Some evidence exists to link both the major psychotic disturbances with some type of disturbance of monoaminergic function.

The monoamine hypothesis of affective disorder

While Parkinsonism was early recognized as a side effect of reserpine therapy, it was soon reported that depression was also a common occurrence in patients receiving reserpine as a treatment for hypertension, and was commoner with higher doses. The incidence of depression in such patients may be as high as 15 per cent, which is well above the expectation of the disease in the general population, and the features of the disorder after reserpine probably do not differ in any major respect from endogenous depression occurring spontaneously. Following the discovery that reserpine depletes the brain of monoamines, the hypothesis was formulated that the ability to provoke depression and to deplete amines are related. The theory is strengthened by observations that drugs such as tetrabenazine and α-methyl-dopa, which also interfere with central monoaminergic mechanisms, are also liable to provoke depression.

The monoamine hypothesis was originally formulated with respect to catecholamines and in the following form: 'that some, if not all, depressions are associated with an absolute or relative decrease in catecholamines, particularly norepinephrine, available at central adrenergic receptor sites'. However, since reserpine and tetrabenazine deplete 5-hydroxytryptamine as well as the catecholamines, and since α-methy-dopa also interferes with 5-hydroxytryptamine synthesis, it

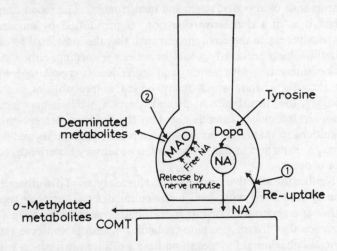

Fig 29. Postulated site of action of the two groups of antidepressant drugs on noradrenaline-containing neurones: (1) iminodibenzyl ('tricyclic') compounds: (2) MAO inhibitors. COMT, catechol-o-methyltransferase; MAO, monoamine oxidase; NA, noradrenaline

seems equally plausible to suggest that some depressions may be associated with a functional deficit of 5-hydroxytryptamine, or of both noradrenaline *and* 5-hydroxytryptamine.

On the basis of the theory that a deficit of one or other monoamine is associated with depression, a plausible explanation of the mode of action of the two main groups of 'antidepressant' drugs can be formulated (Fig. 29): (1) *the monoamine oxidase inhibitors* interfere with the intraneuronal enzymes which dispose of excess amines within the neuronal cytoplasm. This action allows increased concentrations of the amines to accumulate and may thus make humoral transmission more effective; (2) the iminodibenzyl compounds (the '*tricyclic antidepressants*') are effective inhibitors of the re-uptake process into monoamine nerve terminals. By this action they may possibly interfere with the disposal of the neurotransmitter at the site of action, and thus potentiate, and possibly restore towards normal, neural transmission.

Both the monoamine oxidase inhibitors and the more commonly used iminodibenzyl compounds exert actions on both noradrenaline and 5-hydroxytryptamine mechanisms and their therapeutic efficacy, which (particularly in the case of the monoamine oxidase inhibitors) is not striking, cannot be used to support a hypothesis that one rather than the other amine is disturbed in any particular type of depression. Other more direct methods of investigation, including estimation of urinary and c.s.f. (cerebrospinal fluid) metabolites and investigations on post mortem brains have not yet provided unequivocal evidence for either version of the monoamine hypothesis of the affective disorders.

Amphetamine psychosis and schizophrenia

A chemical analogue of the types of disturbance observed in the schizophrenic disorders has been sought by comparing the phenomenology of these disorders with that seen after administration of hallucinogenic drugs such as mescaline and LSD. The mode of action of these agents is very poorly understood and it is clear that the clinical features of the schizophrenias differ considerably from those seen in the 'toxic psychoses' induced by the hallucinogens. A much closer relationship exists, however, between the paranoid psychoses which are seen following ingestion of relatively large doses of the amphetamines and the types of hallucination and thought disorder observed in the paranoid (but probably not other) types of schizophrenia.

It has been argued that the amphetamine psychosis is an idiosyncratic reaction occurring in predisposed individuals, or that it may be a response to the prolonged insomnia produced by the drug. Both explanations can be discounted, however, since it has been shown that the pattern of psychosis can be reliably provoked in normal individuals, and before significant loss of sleep has occurred. This suggests that the chemical disturbance induced by the drug is at the basis of the psychosis. Animal experiments indicate that the amphetamines, which in structure resemble dopamine but lack the ring hydroxl groups, are potent releasers of catecholamines from the nerve endings. The particular behavioural syndrome provoked in animals by these drugs has been closely studied and is very likely to be associated with an increased release of dopamine in the brain.

It is therefore argued that some similar disturbance, i.e. an inappropriate overactivity, of catecholamine mechanisms, may underlie certain schizophrenic states, and it is particularly interesting that the phenothiazine group of drugs, which are the most effective agents in the schizophrenias, are relatively selective blockers of the abnormal animal behaviours induced by the amphetamines. The view that the 'extrapyramidal' side effects of the phenothiazine drugs are essential for their therapeutic effects has been discounted in recent years. However, the antipschyotic effects of the phenothiazine and other groups of drugs effective in schizophrenia are closely related to their ability to block the dopamine receptor. Some such drugs possess two isomeric forms, and it has been shown that in this case only the isomer with dopamine-receptor blocking activity has therapeutic efficacy.

These findings suggest, that in some forms of schizophrenia there might be overactivity of dopaminergic mechanisms. However, studies on c.s.f. levels of the dopamine metabolite homo-vanillic acid (HVA) and on HVA and other metabolites of dopamine in post-mortem brain from patients with schizophrenia reveal no evidence of increased dopamine turnover. From post-mortem studies there is evidence for increased numbers of dopamine receptors. It seems possible in some cases the primary change in schizophrenia may be a supersensitivity of the dopamine receptor.

FURTHER READING

Crow T J Catecholamine-containing neurones and electrical self-stimulation: I and II. Psychological Medicine 2 (1972): 66, / 3 (1973): 414

Crow T J 1980 Molecular pathology of schizophrenia: more than one disease process? British Medical Journal 280: 66

Griffith J D, Cavanaugh J, Held J, Oates J A 1972 Dextroamphetamine: evaluation of psychotomimetic properties in man. Archives of General Psychiatry 26: 97

Hornykiewicz O 1973 Dopamine in the basal ganglia. British Medical Bulletin 29: 172

Johnstone E C, Crow T J, Frith C D, Carney M W P, Price J S 1978 Mechanism of the antipsychotic effect in the treatment of acute schizophrenia. Lancet i: 848

Kety S S, Schildkraut J J 1967 Biogenic amines and emotion. Science, New York 156: 21

Munkvad I, Pakkenberg H, Randrup A 1968 Aminergic systems in basal ganglia associated with stereotyped hyperactive behaviour and catalepsy. Brain, Behaviour, Evolution 1: 89

Owen F, Cross A J, Crow T J, Longden A, Poulter M, Riley G J 1978 Increased dopamine receptor sensitivity in schizophrenia. Lancet ii: 223

Schildkraut J J 1965 The catecholamine hypothesis of affective disorders: a review of supporting evidence. American Journal of Psychiatry 122: 509

Ungerstedt U 1971 Stereotaxic mapping of the monamine pathways in the rat brain. Acta physiologica scandinavica 367: suppl. 1

Vogt M 1969 Release from brain tissue of compounds with possible transmitter functions. British Journal of Pharmacology 37: 325

Index

CHURCHILL LIVINGSTONE
MEDICAL TEXTS

Epidemiology in Medical Practice
Second edition
D. J. P. Barker and G. Rose

Pain: its Nature, Analysis and Treatment
Michael R. Bond

Essentials of Dermatology
J. L. Burton

An Introduction to Clinical Rheumatology
Second edition
William Carson Dick

Elements of Medical Genetics
Fifth edition
Alan E. H. Emery

A Concise Textbook of Gastroenterology
Second edition
M. J. S. Langman

Tumours: Basic Principles and Clinical Aspects
Christopher Louis

Nutrition and its Disorders
Third edition
Donald S. McLaren

The Essentials of Neuroanatomy
Third edition
G. A. G. Mitchell and D. Mayor

Clinical Bacteriology
P. W. Ross

Sexually Transmitted Diseases
Third edition
C. B. S. Schofield

Respiratory Medicine
Second edition
Malcolm Schonell

An Introduction to General Pathology
Second edition
W. G. Spector

Child Psychiatry for Students
Second edition
Frederick H. Stone and Cyrille Koupernik

Introduction to Clinical Endocrinology
Second edition
John A. Thomson

Notes on Medical Virology
Sixth edition
Morag C. Timbury

Clinical Pharmacology
Third edition
P. Turner and A. Richens

Immunology: an Outline for Students of Medicine and Biology
Fourth edition
D. M. Weir

Clinical Thinking and Practice: Diagnosis and Decision in Patient Care
H. J. Wright and D. B. MacAdam

LIVINGSTONE MEDICAL TEXTS
Geriatric Medicine for Students
J. C. Brocklehurst and T. Hanley

Introduction to Clinical Examination
Second edition
Edited by John Macleod

An Introduction to Primary Medical Care
David Morrell

Urology and Renal Medicine
Second edition
J. B. Newman and J. J. B. Petrie

Psychological Medicine for Students
John Pollitt

Cardiology for Students
Max Zoob